The Autistic Spectrum

The Autistic Spectrum

*A Parents' Guide
to Understanding
and Helping
Your Child*

LORNA WING, M.D.

FOREWORD BY
**PROFESSORS AMI KLIN &
FRED VOLKMAR**

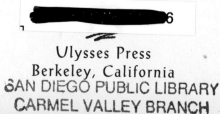

Ulysses Press
Berkeley, California

Published by: Ulysses Press
P.O. Box 3440
Berkeley, CA 94703
www.ulyssespress.com

Library of Congress Catalog Card Number: 00-109473
ISBN: 1-56975-257-5

First published in hardback in Great Britain by Constable and Company, Limited

Printed in Canada by Transcontinental Printing

10 9 8 7 6 5 4 3 2

Editorial and production staff: Leslie Henriques, Steven Zah Schwartz, Lynette Ubois, Demetra Markis, Marin Van Young, Lily Chou, Lisa Kester
Design: Leslie Henriques, Sarah Levin
Cover Photography: Michelle and Phil Abrams
Indexer: Sayre Van Young
U.S. Research: Sanno Zack

Distributed in the United States by Publishers Group West

For Susan

Table of Contents

Foreword

Drawing on a rich history of personal involvement, effective clinical research and dedicated advocacy work, Dr. Lorna Wing's book is a treasure to parents and required reading for any student, educator or mental health professional serving individuals with autism and their families. With characteristic honesty and straightforward prose, combined with a balanced and empirical stance, Dr. Wing navigates us effortlessly through the complexities of clinical work and current research. More importantly, no practical aspect of care is neglected. It takes someone like Lorna Wing to know that sometimes the most fierce battles in autism are waged around mundane daily routines. Although not always glamorous, this knowledge is certainly crucial.

The central role Dr. Wing has played in making society more aware of the needs of individuals with autism and their families may not be well known to readers outside of Britain. A formidable advocate, she was one of a small number of parents in the U.K. and U.S. who was not satisfied with the neglect that had been bestowed upon children with autism. These parents created schools, parent support organizations, fierce lobbying groups, and effective community campaigns that laid the foundations for today's growing network of resources for children, adolescents and adults with autism and their families. To those of us who have worked with Dr. Wing, this love always appeared to come above all else, and her friends and colleagues at the National Autistic Society in Britain have more than one anecdote to color the story of how services for those with autism came into being in the U.K.

This book also reflects Lorna Wing's unique gift for combining clinical observation and research. Over the past three decades, her work has helped change the climate in which children with autism, and their families, are seen and understood. Her epidemiological studies rescued autism from earlier theories that blamed parents and helped place it squarely within the field of biomedical study. Her insights into the nature of the psychological deficits in children with autism set the stage for important work that focuses on the derailment of symbolic and conceptual development in this condition. Her schemes for characterizing levels of social disability paved the way to the view of autism as a spectrum of social disorders. And these are only a few examples of her accomplishments. All of these lines of research contributed to a much more complex view of autism, where respect for individuality is crucial, both in research and in clinical services.

Dr. Wing does not have all the answers to the puzzle of autistic spectrum disorders, but she does pose all of the important questions. A scientist once said that we do not have full understanding of a phenomenon until we have a good measure of it. We are still missing such a measure, but thankfully we do not need to wait for one in order to effectively serve individuals with autism and their families. For that purpose, this book is an invaluable guide.

Ami Klin, Ph.D.
Harris Associate Professor

Fred Volkmar, M.D.
Professor

Child Study Center
Yale University
New Haven, CT 06520

Introduction

I wrote the first version of this book in 1970. It was then called *Autistic Children: A Guide for Parents*. The present book has been almost entirely rewritten. In 1970, interest was focused mainly on the so-called typical autistic syndrome, which was defined very narrowly. The theory that autism was caused by a cold, mechanical style of parenting by university-educated, middle-class parents was still strongly held by many professionals. Little was known about outcome in adult life. Since then, a spectrum of disorders that is much wider than "typical autism" has become widely recognized. The fact that the autistic spectrum comprises disorders of development caused by physical dysfunction of the brain is now generally accepted and a great deal is known about the outcome in adult life. There is just as much heated debate as there was in 1970. However, now the scientific searchlight is centered on specifying the criteria for diagnosis, differentiating subgroups that might have different causes or need different methods of treatment, defining the boundaries of the spectrum and examining questions of neuropathology and how it is expressed in psychological mechanisms and overt behavior.

The story behind this evolution of ideas began in 1943, when Leo Kanner published a paper about a number of children referred to his clinic. This small group of children had in common an unusual pattern of behavior that he named "early infantile autism." He gave detailed descriptions of the children's behavior but selected certain features as crucial for diagnosis. These were profound lack of affective (emotional) contact with other people; intense insistence on sameness in their self-chosen, often bizarre and elaborate repetitive routines; mutism or marked abnormality of speech; fascination with and dexterity in manipulating objects; high levels of visuo-spatial skills or rote memory in contrast to learning difficulties in other areas; an attractive, alert, intelligent appearance. Later, Kanner suggested that the first two of these features were sufficient for diagnosis. He also emphasized that the condition was present from birth or began within the first 30 months of life. He believed his syndrome was unique and separate from all other childhood conditions.

In the first decades of the 20th century, the psychoanalytic theories influenced the attitudes of professionals and the public at large. Many people, including Kanner, believed that autism was an emotional, not a physical disorder and that the way the parents had brought up their child had caused all the problems. The effect was disastrous—it exacerbated the parents' distress at having a child with behavior they could not understand, made them feel guilty and damaged any confidence they may have had in their ability to help their child.

My daughter, Susan, was born in 1956. My husband, John, and I were worried about her almost from the time she was born. By 1960 we knew for sure that she had autism in very typical form. It so happened that 1960 saw the start of a marked change in ideas about autism. The work of researchers in Britain and the U.S. was beginning to show that the behavior of children with autism made most sense if viewed as the result of developmental disorders, starting from birth or the early years of childhood. Growing knowledge of brain function pointed to biological causes. John and I were psychiatrists in research concerned with the epidemiology of mental illnesses and mental retardation and we had close colleagues who were working in the field of autistic disorders. This had two major consequences. From the personal point of view, we were able to reject with confidence any suggestion that we had caused our much-wanted and much-loved daughter to be autistic. From the professional point of view we were able to use our experience of autism in our research work.

We helped in the planning of the first study of the prevalence of autism, which was carried out by Victor Lotter in an English county. Lotter concentrated on finding children with typical autism as described by Kanner. He found a rate of 4.5 in every 10,000 children. He noted that almost all of these children had some degree of mental retardation and some had associated conditions suggestive of brain dysfunction.

This study left some important questions unanswered. How many children were there with features of autism but not the full picture? Were these children's needs for care and treatment similar to or different from those with typical autism? What was the relationship of autism to other developmental disorders? Was there really a significant tendency for the parents to be middle-class and university-educated?

In the early 1970s my colleague Judith Gould and I had the opportunity to carry out an epidemiological study of children in a London borough, Camberwell, which we hoped might help answer some of these questions. We examined children born in 1956 through the 1970s who had any kind of physical or psychological disability or abnormality of behavior, however mild or severe. We found we could identify a group with typical Kanner's autism but we also found many others who had features of autistic behavior but who did not precisely fit Kanner's criteria.

Halfway through the study, we became aware of the work of another author that shed light on the clinical pictures we were seeing in some children. In 1944, Hans Asperger, in Austria, had published his first paper on a group of children and adolescents with the pattern of behavior now referred to as Asperger's syndrome. The features he selected as important were as follows: naive, inappropriate social approaches to others; intense circumscribed interest in particular subjects such as railway timetables; good grammar and vocabulary but monotonous speech used for monologues, not two-way conversation; poor motor coordination; level of ability in the

borderline, average or superior range but often with specific learning difficulties in one or two subjects; a marked lack of common
sense. He noted that, although problems were present earlier in development, the parents usually did not observe any abnormality
until after three years or until the children started school. He believed that his syndrome was different from Kanner's autism,
though he admitted there were many similarities.

Asperger published his findings toward the end of World War
II and there was a long delay before papers on the subject appeared in the English literature. It is only in the last 10 to 20 years
that Asperger's work has become well known outside continental
Europe.

In our Camberwell study, we did identify some children who
fit Asperger's descriptions. We now know that if we had had enough
resources to include children from mainstream schools, we would
certainly have found many more with Asperger's syndrome. The
main findings from this study were, first, that Kanner's and Asperger's syndromes are sub-groups among a wide range of disorders
affecting social interaction and communication; many children have
mixtures of features of both syndromes. Second, that these conditions could be associated with any level of intelligence. Third, that
they are sometimes associated with various physical conditions or
other developmental disabilities. Fourth, that parents of children
with typical autism and other autistic disorders come from any
kind of background—there is no middle class bias. Last but not
least, we found that all those with any kind of autistic spectrum
disorder have the same need for a structured, organized environment and daily program.

Later, Christopher Gillberg and his colleagues in Sweden examined children with average or high intelligence attending mainstream schools. He identified a number of children with autistic
features including some fitting Kanner's or Asperger's descriptions.
The results of both these studies strongly supported the hypothesis, which was beginning to be taken seriously, that there was a
very wide spectrum of autistic disorders characterized by the triad

of impairments of social interaction, communication and imagination associated with a narrow range of repetitive activities.

The changes over the years of ideas about autistic disorders are reflected by the two international systems of classifying psychiatric and behavioral disorders. These are the *International Statistical Classification of Diseases and Related Health Problems* (ICD) published by the World Health Organization, and the *Diagnostic and Statistical Manual* (DSM) of the American Psychiatric Association. The first editions of these two publications did not include autism at all. The disorder was not mentioned until the eighth edition of the ICD appeared in 1967. This listed "infantile autism" as a form of schizophrenia. It was not until 1980 that the idea that autism was a developmental disorder and part of a wider range of related conditions appeared in the third edition of the DSM. The current edition of both systems (DSM-IV and ICD-10) include these ideas. The name used in both to cover autism and related conditions is Pervasive Developmental Disorder (PDD). (I prefer the term "autistic spectrum disorder," which I use in this book, because the parents I meet tend to find it easier to understand than PDD.)

Since completing the Camberwell study, I have continued to work in the field of autism. I have examined the manifestations of autistic disorders in adults. I have been particularly interested in problems of diagnosis. After I retired from full-time research, I worked with Judith Gould to set up, for Britain's National Autistic Society, a center for diagnosis and assessment of children and adults with social and communication disorders. We have developed an interview schedule (The Diagnostic Interview for Social and Communication Disorders, known as DISCO), which is designed for clinical assessment of needs as well as diagnosis. I am now a part-time psychiatric consultant to this center and value the regular contact with families from whom I continue to learn so much. For the last two years, my colleagues and I have also been running training courses on diagnosis for professionals in the field.

There has been a steady advance in knowledge about the nature of autistic conditions, although there is still a long way to go.

Despite many claims for the success of different approaches, no curative methods of treatment have been scientifically validated as yet. However, there have been major advances in understanding how to create a suitable environment and a daily program of education, occupation and leisure activities that minimize the disabilities and maximize the potential skills of people with autistic spectrum disorders. Much of the impetus for improving the lives of people with these conditions has come from parents, who joined together with concerned professionals to form voluntary associations to work on behalf of people with autistic disorders. The first groups of this kind began in the 1960s almost simultaneously in the U.S. and the U.K. Parents in many other countries have now followed this lead.

Research and clinical experience have demonstrated the wide range of outcomes in adult life, from total dependence to independence in spite of residual disabilities. Outcome is closely related to level of ability, which can be assessed fairly accurately from about five or six years of age onwards. For parents of the most severely affected children it is hard to be presented with the facts about the future. The writer of a book for parents of children and adults of all ages and all levels of ability is faced with a dilemma; how much of the whole picture should be given? But, even if it were desirable, it is becoming increasingly difficult to hide the truth because of newspaper and magazine articles, books, videos, TV programs and feature films. Most parents do want all the facts, negative as well as positive, so that they can form a realistic plan of action.

My own daughter is severely affected and, as an adult, remains dependent on others, though happy living in a small home designed for people with autistic disorders. John and I are glad that we were told the truth about the severity of her disabilities when she was diagnosed as a young child. It was very painful at the time, but we were able to come to terms with the situation and, seen against the background of her severe problems, each small advance she has made has been a source of deep joy and satisfaction.

My aim in writing this book has been to give a clear, jargon-free account of current ideas on autistic disorders and what parents and professional workers can do to help children and adults who have these conditions. In the first part of the book I describe the features of behavior seen in autistic spectrum disorders at different phases of life, the subgroups found in the spectrum and the problems of making a diagnosis. I discuss the question of the numbers of people affected, the different conditions that can occur together with the spectrum and the various theories concerning causes. In the second part of the book, I consider the effects on the family of having a child with an autistic disorder and I describe positive ways of meeting the challenges. I also outline the roles of professional workers and of the educational, social and health services that become involved.

On a different note altogether, in addition to all the other changes since the first version of this book, the dreaded Political Correctness has cast a long shadow and I have conformed. In the first edition, the term "autistic children" was used, doctors, psychologists and autistic children were referred to as "he," and teachers were always "she." Now, these automatic assumptions seem wrong, even to one not in the forefront of the PC movement. The current terms are "children/adults with autism/autistic spectrum disorders." The pronouns "they, them and their" are used regardless of singular or plural in order to avoid ascribing gender whenever possible. As in 1970, I have referred throughout to "parents" in the plural. I am now conscious of the growing number of single parents who have children with autistic disorders. Please read references to parents in the plural to mean one parent alone or together with a partner.

Another difference from 1970 is that many books on autistic disorders are now available, some of which are in the reading list at the end of this book. Most deal with particular aspects of the subject. This book is a general introduction, intended to lead on to more specialized texts. It fills a particular niche because my dual role as parent of a grown-up daughter with autism and a professional with research and clinical experience provides an insight that cannot be obtained from any one of these viewpoints alone. Perhaps this book will enable parents and professionals to understand each other a little better and thereby increase the help that each can give to children and adults with autistic spectrum disorders.

People with autistic disorders have the same basic patterns of behavior wherever they live. When parents from different countries meet, cultural barriers melt away and common experiences are shared. The original version of this book is translated into different languages (the latest being Chinese) and has been read by parents and professionals all over the world. I hope that this new book will transcend barriers the same way the first one did.

PART I

Description of Autistic Spectrum Disorders

CHAPTER 1

The Nature of Autistic Spectrum Disorders

Once it was recognized that autistic behavior was a result of problems of development, interest focused on which skills were not developing properly. In order for a baby to become a fully functioning and independent adult, many different abilities have to appear at the appropriate stages and then grow in complexity. At first, many of us working in this field believed that autistic behavior resulted from disorders of language development. This appeared plausible because so many of the children had delayed and deviant language or none at all. It seemed that if understanding and use of spoken speech and communication by gestures were all affected, this would account for autistic behavior. At that time, it was hoped that overcoming these specific language problems by some alternative method of communication would produce major improvement. This theory had to be rejected when it was found that some children and adults with autistic spectrum disorders developed good grammar and vocabularies and even used some gestures, though they still had autistic behavior.

A clue to the nature of autism came from accounts of the behavior of babies as remembered by their parents. In infants who are later diagnosed as having autistic disorders, lack of interest in social interaction is often present from very early on, well before the time speech develops. Studies of normal early development show that there is a built-in interest in the sight and sound of other human beings, especially, at first, the mother or other primary caretaker. There is also a drive to communicate in every possible way, through bodily movements and baby noises, before speech begins, and to respond to communications from others. These built-in "instincts" can be seen very early in the first year.

In the second year, another aspect of the social skills should begin to emerge—that is, imagination. The child starts to play with toys, first for the simple sensations, then to use them for their obvious purposes, and then for pretend games. The child becomes able to pretend that one object represents another—a box is a bed for a baby doll, or a row of chairs is a bus. Later, children play together and develop complex imaginative games. Imagination enables all kinds of skills to be practiced. In particular, it enables a child to pretend to be other people and take on their roles in social play. Playing games of this kind depends upon the child having developed the knowledge, built-in but taking time to emerge, that other people have thought and feelings—the so-called "Theory of Mind." When this has emerged, pretend games help to improve skill in understanding other people that is necessary for integration into social life.

These abilities are just as dependent upon brain function as all other developmental skills. They are absent or severely impaired in children with autism. In the study in Camberwell, described in the introduction, we found that all the children with "autistic features," whether they fit Kanner's or Asperger's descriptions or had bits and pieces of both, had in common absence or impairments of social interaction, communication and development of imagination. They also all had a narrow, rigid, repetitive pattern of activities and interests. The three impairments (referred to as the "triad") and the repetitive activities were shown in a wide variety of ways, but the underlying similarities were recognizable.

There can be no doubt that a yet more fundamental impairment of psychological function underlies the triad. It is likely that there is an inability to put together all kinds of information derived from past memories and present events, to make sense of experiences, to predict what is likely to happen in the future and to make plans. People with autistic disorders do not make sense of the world and find it hard to learn from experience. They find it difficult to organize themselves in time and in space. Uta Frith wrote that they lacked what she called a "drive for central coherence." The more complex the incoming information, the harder it is for an individual with an autistic disorder to understand. Human beings are extremely complicated and variable in their speech, movements and reactions, so it is not surprising that impairment of social interaction is a major feature of autistic disorders.

It is possible that, at an even deeper level, there is a disturbance of the normal built-in system for assigning different degrees of emotional significance to different experiences. There are various theories concerning how the brain originally assigns emotional value to the biological necessities for survival and reproduction and then, building on these, develops over the years a complex system of values related to the culture in which the individual lives. Whatever the neural mechanisms, it appears that people with autistic disorders are impaired in their ability to distinguish between the important and the trivial. In some of the young children there is indifference even to food. In all those affected, the lack of interest in others is a defining feature. Coupled with this is the idiosyncratic fascination for specific objects or experiences that appear trivial and meaningless to others.

One day we may have tests that demonstrate the nature of the basic problems. For the present, recognizing autistic spectrum disorders has to depend on detecting the triad of impairments because the three impairments can be identified from knowledge of an individual's development and behavior.

CHAPTER 2

Making a Diagnosis

Despite the fact that the existence of autistic disorders has become much more widely known, there are still difficulties surrounding diagnosis. Most of the children look physically normal. Minor congenital abnormalities, which are reported to be common in the children, do not adversely affect their appearance, which is often very attractive, not the least because of the quality of mysterious remoteness. There are no tests yet developed that can be used to make a definitive diagnosis of autism nor any that can tell the difference between sub-groups with autistic disorders. Blood tests, X-rays, brain scans, electroencephalograms (records of the electrical waves from the brain) and other physical examinations cannot give a positive answer to the question, "Does this child have an autistic disorder?" Psychological examinations, including the recently developed "Theory of Mind" tests (see Chapter 6), though helpful in other ways, cannot be used to confirm or refute the presence of an autistic spectrum disorder. There is reason to hope that useful tests will be found but we do not have them at the present time.

In this situation, diagnosis is made by recognizing patterns of behavior present from early in life. All systems for diagnoses that have been suggested, including the ICD and DSM, agree that the impairments of social interaction, communication and imagination and the rigid, repetitive pattern of activities are crucial diagnostic features. Despite this fundamental accord, disagreements over diagnosis of individual children and adults arise for many reasons, including the following.

1. The impairments can be shown in many different ways, some of which are subtle and not easy to recognize.

2. Autistic spectrum disorders can occur together with any level of general intelligence, from profound disability to well above average.

3. They can occur together with any other physical disability or developmental disorder. Epileptic seizures are particularly common.

4. Changes in the behavior pattern can occur with increasing age.

5. Behavior can vary according to the environment. It is often worse at home where parents have many competing demands for their attention than it is at a well-organized school or clinic.

6. Behavior can vary depending on the person the child or adult is with. It is always better with an adult who is experienced in working with autistic disorders than it is with inexperienced people or in unstructured groups. Some adults who are high-functioning, including those with the pattern described by Asperger, may show no signs of their impairments in one-to-one situations, including interviews with a psychiatrist. The problems are revealed in their life history, especially in the way they cope with events they find stressful.

7. Education often affects the behavior pattern.

8. Each individual's own personality shines through and influences their behavior.

Diagnosis depends on compiling a personal history that links together all the available information. Ideally, the history from infancy and a description of the present behavior should be collected systematically by interview with the parents. A schedule of questions designed to diagnose autistic spectrum disorders should be used so that all important details are covered. In addition, the behavior of the individual should be observed and a range of psychological tests should be given. All this takes time to complete—at least two to three hours for the interview alone. If the procedure is rushed and the right questions are not asked the diagnosis can be missed.

Sub-groups of Autistic Spectrum Disorders

When an autistic disorder is diagnosed, there is the further problem of deciding which sub-group in the spectrum the individual belongs to. Now that the term Asperger's syndrome is being used more widely, parents and professional workers want to know how it differs from other forms of autism. Since Asperger's group, unlike Kanner's, includes mostly those with average or high levels of ability, the main question is how to tell Asperger's syndrome from high-functioning Kanner's autism. There is no simple answer. It is possible to find some individuals who have all the features described by Kanner and others who fit Asperger's syndrome perfectly. However, there are many who fit neither of these syndromes precisely, having mixtures of features of both. Furthermore, it is quite common to find people who had the behavior typical of Kanner's syndrome in early childhood who change with age until, by adolescence, they behave just like someone with Asperger's syndrome.

In the latest editions of the ICD and DSM classification systems, Asperger's syndrome is distinguished from other autistic disorders by having no delay in onset of speech and other aspects of the development of adaptive skills. The difficulty with this is that many people who, by adolescence, have the behavior Asperger described, did have developmental delays, including later speaking.

ICD-10 also includes "atypical autism" diagnosed on either insufficient features for typical autism, or onset after three years, or both. In DSM-IV this would be classified as "other pervasive developmental disorder." Parents find these diagnoses unhelpful. Such children present the same disturbances of behavior and have the same needs as those with typical autism. It is particularly distressing if the label "atypical" is used as an excuse to exclude a child from appropriate educational services.

ICD-10 and DSM-IV also include a diagnosis of "childhood disintegrative disorder." In this, development is said to be normal up to two years and then there is loss of skills in at least two of the following areas: language; play; social skills or adaptive behavior; bowel or bladder control; motor skills. This diagnosis is also a source of confusion. A substantial minority of children with autistic disorders begin to say words around one year and then stop speaking. Some start again later and some do not. Around the time they cease to speak they often become more socially withdrawn and perhaps lose the interest they had in manipulating toys. The vast majority of these children, whether or not they begin to speak again, have clinical pictures that cannot be distinguished from others with autistic disorders who did not show a temporary or permanent loss of skills in their second or third year. The course and prognosis are the same as with other autistic disorders of comparable severity.

The word "disintegrative" suggests a downhill course and some parents of children given this diagnosis expect the child to become progressively more disabled. Very rarely, this does happen because the child concerned has a physical condition affecting the brain that is progressive. The autistic pattern of behavior is seen during one stage of this progression. These conditions need to be identified and separated from the usual autistic spectrum disorders. They alone merit the label "disintegrative."

Elizabeth Newson described a pattern of behavior in children that she called "pathological demand avoidance" (PDA) syndrome. The children concerned have speech but use this to distract their teacher or caretaker so they can avoid doing any task. Once again, the problem is that children who have any kind of autistic spectrum disorder can show this type of behavior.

Some workers are studying whether autistic disorders associated with high levels of ability have other specific differences from those associated with varying degrees of generalized learning difficulties. There certainly are differences but it is not clear if they are due only to differing severity of the disabilities or if there are differences in the nature of the impairments underlying the clinical pictures.

Attempts to delineate specific sub-groups of autistic spectrum disorders are confounded by the considerable overlap among the suggested syndromes. The clinical picture of every type of autistic disorder is made up of a large number of features. In clinical practice the more you see of these conditions, the more it appears that any combination of the features is possible. Some combinations are more likely than others but there are no absolute rules. The boundaries are always difficult to define.

For all these reasons, from the point of view of helping the person concerned, spending time on assigning them to a sub-group is of little value. The main clinical task is to decide if they have an autistic spectrum disorder and then to assess their pattern of abilities. The demands of research are different from those of clinical work and investigators may reasonably choose to examine whether specific, separate sub-groups can be found among the autism spectrum disorders. The important point is to separate the need to help individuals from the demands of research.

CHAPTER 3

The Behavior of Children
with Autistic Spectrum Disorders

Each individual with an autistic spectrum disorder is different from every other so these descriptions should be taken as a general guide and not as an exact specification for diagnosis. Nevertheless, the common problems affecting social interaction, communication and imagination and the repetitive behavior can be recognized behind all the variations.

Many, perhaps most, children with autistic disorders show signs of their social and communication problems from early infancy. But, because they cannot move around, the range of behavior possible for a baby is limited. For this reason, at this stage the signs of the impairments are not obvious and are easily missed by parents. It is not until the child begins to walk independently that the full extent of autistic behavior can emerge.

Behavior in Babies

Because diagnosis is rarely made before two years of age at the earliest, the details of behavior in babyhood have been collected from the memories of parents of older children.

Some babies who later show autistic behavior appear to develop normally for a time and their parents do not notice anything unusual in the first year or so. However, for many, perhaps most of these, careful, systematic questioning shows that there were unusual aspects of behavior even in the first year. Other babies gave their parents cause for concern almost from birth. Sometimes mothers say that they felt something was wrong within the first few days, but they usually cannot tell why they had this feeling. Feeding problems are fairly common and some of the babies do not suck well.

There seem to be three kinds of babies who have autistic disorders. The majority tend to be placid and undemanding, content to lie quietly in their cribs all day. Sometimes mothers feel that a child of this kind does not know whether he or she is hungry because they do not cry to be fed. In infancy, they are said to be "angel babies" but parents tend to become concerned as time goes on and the babies do not become more active or sociable. In contrast, a minority scream a great deal both day and night and cannot be comforted or soothed. There are also some babies who are later diagnosed as autistic who fit neither of these descriptions and whose behavior pattern, viewed retrospectively, seemed to show no unusual features.

The babies may dislike any interference such as diaper changing, dressing and washing. They may not lift their arms or make themselves ready to be picked up. When held they tend not to snuggle down comfortably in their mother's arms and, later on, may not grip with their hands and knees if carried piggyback. Some babies are fascinated by lights, or by anything that shines, twinkles or spins. An intense interest in the visual stimuli from the television set may appear very early, as may fascination with music. On the other hand, the babies seem uninterested in things that catch the attention of other babies as they grow and develop. Typically, they do not lean out of their strollers in eager curiosity to look at people and animals and the passing scene, nor do they try to attract their mother's attention to these things by pointing and making eye contact. A recent study by Simon Baron-Cohen and colleagues has shown that, if this behavior is absent at 18 months of age, it is very likely indeed that the child is autistic. Some do point to one or a few specific things that interest them but are not concerned to share the enjoyment. Some do not begin to point until long past infancy, if at all. Babies may smile when tickled, cuddled or bounced up and down, but not when looking at someone's face. They may not join in by copying the parents' actions in baby games such as peek-a-boo or patty-cake.

Babies with autistic disorders often smile, cut their teeth, sit up, crawl and walk at the usual ages and gain weight normally, once early feeding problems have passed. Sometimes the motor milestones are delayed, especially in those who later fit Asperger's descriptions or those who have other disabilities affecting motor development. They may not bother to sit up even when able to, apparently because the world is of little interest. A number of the children stand up and walk holding on to the furniture at the right time, but may be reluctant to let go and walk without support until many months after the usual age. There are some stories of young children who crawled or shuffled everywhere until two or more years of age and then suddenly stood up and walked and ran without any previous practice.

Babbling tends to be limited in quantity and poor in quality and usually does not develop the intonation pattern and range of sounds of ordinary speech, which normally begins around the end of the first year.

Behavior Diagnostic of Autism Spectrum Disorders

For the majority of children with autistic disorders, parents become aware of problems gradually. They often begin to worry in the second year if the child is not talking or if the behavior pattern is different from that of other children of the same age. If the child has a high level of skill in some areas parents may not become concerned until the third year or even later. In a minority, development appears to the parents to be proceeding normally, then a marked change in behavior occurs over a few weeks or months, perhaps with regression in some skills, particularly speech. In both types of onset, the behavior diagnostic of an autistic spectrum disorder emerges sooner or later in the pre-school years.

I shall start by describing the triad of social, communication and imagination impairments and the repetitive behavior that are crucial for diagnosis and then go on to the other features that are often seen.

Impairments of Social Interaction

This is shown in different ways. It is easiest to describe the varieties by grouping them into four main types, although there is no sharp cut-off between them.

The Aloof Group

This is probably the single most common type of social impairment in young children and is seen most clearly at this stage. In some it continues throughout life, though others do change as they grow older.

Those who are socially aloof behave as though other people do not exist. They do not come when they are called, they do not respond if you speak to them, their faces may be empty of expression except when they experience the extremes of anger, distress or joy, they look through or past you, just occasionally giving you a quick sideways glance, they may pull away if you touch them, they do not put their arms around you if you cuddle them and they may walk past you (or over you, if you are sitting on the floor) without pausing in their stride.

If they want something they cannot reach they grab you by the back of your hand or arm, not placing their hand inside yours or looking up at you, and pull you along to use your hand to reach the object they desire or to carry out an action for them such as turning the handle of a door. Once the object is obtained, you are ignored again.

They show no interest or sympathy if you are in pain or distress. They seem cut off, in a world of their own, completely absorbed in their own aimless activities. However, as children, most of them do respond to rough-and-tumble play. When tickled, swung around, rolled on the floor or chased around they may laugh with delight and show great pleasure. They may even look into your eyes and indicate that they want you to continue. In these situations, the children seem happy and sociable, as if nothing is wrong. The moment the game is finished the child becomes aloof once more.

In childhood, the social impairment is particularly noticeable in contrast to other children of the same age. In normal development, interest in other children is evident very early on, well before school age. Young children with autistic disorders in the aloof group are indifferent to or alarmed by their companions in play group or nursery school. Even if they will accept their sisters or brothers, they do not interact with children outside the family. The adults who continue to be aloof have no interest in their peers. If they want something they approach whoever is in charge, though how, despite their social impairments, they unerringly identify the senior person is an unsolved mystery.

THE PASSIVE GROUP

This is the least common type of social impairment. These children or adults are not completely cut off from others. They accept social approaches and do not move away from others, but they do not initiate social interaction. They may have poor eye contact, like the aloof group, but are more likely to meet other people's gaze when reminded to do so. Because, during childhood, they are amenable and willing to do as they are told, other children are often happy to involve them in their play. A passive child makes an ideal baby in a game of mothers and fathers or a patient in a pretend hospital. The problem is that when the game changes, the passive child may be left behind because there is no suitable role for them.

In general, children and adults of this kind have the least behavior problems of any with autistic disorders. However, some change markedly in adolescence and become disturbed in behavior.

THE "ACTIVE BUT ODD" GROUP

I first described this group in a paper written in 1979. Ever since then I have tried to think of a name that sounds better but without success. "Active but odd" describes them precisely and many people now use the term.

Children and adults of this kind make active approaches to other people, usually those in charge rather than their age peers, but do so in a peculiar one-sided fashion to make demands or to go and on about their own concerns. They pay no attention to the feelings or needs of the people they talk to. Some have poor eye contact but the problem is usually timing of making and breaking eye contact rather than avoidance. They often stare too long and hard when talking to, or rather at, others. Their approaches can include physically holding or hugging the other person, often much too tightly. They can become difficult and aggressive if they are not given the attention they demand. In childhood, they may ignore children of their own age or else behave aggressively toward them.

This group tends to present particular diagnostic problems because the active social approaches cover up the fact that they have no real understanding of how to interact socially with other people.

THE OVER-FORMAL, STILTED GROUP

This pattern of behavior is not seen until later adolescence and adult life. It develops in those who are the most able and have a good level of language. They are excessively polite and formal in their behavior. They try very hard to behave well and cope by sticking rigidly to the rules of social interaction. They do not really understand these rules and have special difficulty with adapting to the subtle differences in behavior expected in different situations and the changes that occur over time. They can make mistakes because of this lack of true understanding. One young man was as distantly polite to his family as he was to strangers. However, he wished to have a girlfriend and, after reading a magazine article about the need to be positive and seize the initiative, he approached a girl he did not know and asked her very politely if he could kiss her.

The lack of understanding of other people's thoughts and feelings is evident in all the different sub-groups, even when there is the desire to be kind and helpful.

Impairments of Communications

All children and adults with autistic disorders have problems with *communication*. Their *language* (that is grammar, vocabulary, even the ability to define the meanings of single words) may or may not be impaired. The problem lies with the way they use whatever language they do have.

Using Speech

Delay and abnormality in development of speech are very common and Kanner considered them to be an essential part of his syndrome. The difficulties vary in severity. Some children, perhaps one in four or five of all those with autistic spectrum disorders, never speak and remain mute all their lives. Some of these are able to produce accurate copies of animal or mechanical noises and perhaps a single word once in a blue moon but do not progress beyond this.

The rest do develop speech, though many begin much later than normal. They often start by repeating words spoken by other people, especially the last word or the last few words of a sentence. The exact accent and intonation of the speaker may be copied. The repetition of words may have little meaning for the child and this empty echoing, like a parrot, is called "echolalia." Some children repeat words or phrases they have heard in the past and this is called "delayed echolalia." Such phrases may be used appropriately in some situations to ask for things they want. Because the child is copying the exact words of the speaker, they reverse the pronouns, for example, asking for a drink by saying "Do you want juice?" with the intonation of a question because this is what they have heard many times when given a drink.

A child may always use the same phrase or sentence in a particular situation because that was how it was first heard. The association of the phrase with the situation may be completely arbitrary. Kanner gave the example of a boy who said "Peter eater" whenever he saw anything that looked like a saucepan because his mother had been reciting "Peter, Peter, pumpkin eater" when she had accidentally dropped a saucepan. This idiosyncratic way of using words sounds very odd to strangers though parents can usually work out the reasons why the child has latched on to the phrase.

Some children never pass the stage of echoed speech but others move on to the next phase, when they begin to say some words and phrases they work out for themselves. At first a child will name things that they want, such as "candy," "drink," "ice cream." They may then, after months or years, go on to use spontaneous phrases, which may be produced with painful effort, often with mistakes in grammar and word meanings.

As if they are learning a foreign language, the children may find difficulty with the little linking words such as "in," "on," "under," "before" and "because." They may leave them out altogether, saying for example "want dinner," "go car shops." Later on they may put them in sentences but use them incorrectly, as in "put cup in table," "sit from chair." One particular mistake the children make is to confuse two words that are opposite in meaning, or else to use one word of the pair for both its true and its opposite meaning. Thus "switch on light" may be a request to switch the light on or off depending on the circumstances. Often one can see that the child is using the word "on" to say "do something appropriate to the light" and that the precise meaning of "on" and "off" has not been grasped. Similarly, words that usually occur in pairs can be confused. "Brush" may be called "comb," or "sock" may be called "shoe." Even "Mommy" and "Daddy" may be mis-named although the child's behavior clearly shows that they differentiate between their parents.

Some children retain these abnormalities of speech into adult life. Others improve in their speech and some, sooner or later, develop good grammar and a large vocabulary. Some have apparently normal speech without any early delay, especially those who, as adolescents and adults, fit the description given by Asperger of his syndrome. But, even those who do appear to have normal language have a range of subtle problems. There are some who, despite having a good vocabulary, speak very little. Others talk at length but tend not to use colloquial expressions, so that their speech sounds old-fashioned and pedantic. If asked a question they give full replies, often providing far more detail than is needed. One young man was asked in a psychological test why police were needed. He launched into the history of the police, starting with Sir Robert Peel. Some love dictionaries and encyclopedias and this is evident in their speech. It has been said that the speech of a person of this kind is similar to that of a computer translating from a foreign language, like the boy who asked his mother, "May I extract a cookie from the container?" and another who after being given a cup of tea said, "I wish to thank you for the hospitality you have extended to me this afternoon."

The content of the speech of those children and adults who can talk is repetitive and not conversational. They may go on and on asking the same questions regardless of the answers or deliver a monologue on their special interests regardless of the response of the audience. Some adults have learned that such repetitive talking is not socially acceptable and try not to do it but, given the slightest opportunity, they cannot resist returning to their favorite themes.

UNDERSTANDING SPEECH

The level of understanding varies as widely as the use of speech. Some children and adults understand no spoken speech and do not respond when spoken to. They may appear to comprehend more than they really do because they use their eyes to pick up clues to situations.

Most do have some understanding. This may be limited to names of familiar objects or simple instructions in context, such as "Give me your cup" or "Come and have your milk." It can be difficult to know how much understanding there is of the words and how much is guessed from the situation. If the child or adult can be sent out of the room to get one or two objects it is more obvious that they comprehend the words. One source of confusion is the lack of flexibility in word meaning. Difficulties can arise if objects have more than one name. One child had learned that the dog's food was served on "Candy's plate." One day she was asked to give Candy her food in her bowl. The child looked puzzled for a moment, then put the dog's food into the bowl used for washing the dishes.

It is easy to imagine their problems over words that sound the same but have different meanings. For example, a mother said to her daughter, "I'll meet you after dinner." This was heard by her son with an autistic disorder, who then said, "Have meat for dinner" with an expression of pleasure at having understood something at last. This example also illustrates another problem—that is, the tendency to react to one or two words in a sentence and to ignore the rest. One little girl was asked to "Bring Mommy the pullover on the chair in your bedroom." The child trotted upstairs and after several minutes staggered in with the chair.

A major characteristic of people with autistic disorders, however good their language seems to be, is their literal interpretation. One boy was told to "Dry the teapot on the outside, not the inside" and promptly took it out into the garden to wipe it dry. One has to beware of using sayings such as "crying your eyes out" or "have you lost your tongue" because these can be taken at face value and cause distress or even terror. Even people who seem to understand well can make all kinds of mistakes. A man who could travel by himself bought a travel card for the first time. On it was written "valid for travel until midnight." He returned home exhausted having been traveling on the subway until midnight because he thought the words on the card were an absolute instruction. An invitation to a person with autism to "call in and see me again when you are passing," which is said merely for politeness, can lead to many unwanted, lengthy visits at inappropriate times. Children with autistic disorders react badly to verbal teasing because, if they have some understanding, they take it seriously. They also have little or no understanding of jokes that depend on verbal ambiguity. They may try to tell jokes but do not know why they are funny or else they invent jokes that have no point at all. They know that telling funny stories is what people do but they do not understand why.

The most able people with autistic disorders, by the time they are adults, seem to have good understanding and use of complex speech in relation to the subjects that interest them. They can still make elementary mistakes and often seem to understand long, obscure words but be confused by the simplest everyday ones.

Intonation and Voice Control

The great majority of people with autistic disorders have odd intonation, which may be monotonous or inappropriate in inflection.
They have problems in controlling the volume of their speech,
which may be too loud or, less commonly, too quiet. The voice may
have an odd, mechanical, robot-like quality. These difficulties are
more obvious with spontaneous than echoed speech. Improvement
may occur with increasing age.

Some occasionally use a "special" voice, different from their
ordinary one. This may be a copy of something they have heard but
sometimes seems to be an attempt to try out different sounds. When
they do speak, many of the children and adults enunciate words
clearly, although some have varying degrees of difficulty in this aspect of speech.

Using and Understanding Non-verbal Communication

Normally, people communicate with each other in many ways
other than speaking. They use gestures, facial expressions and bodily movements to accompany speech. In a foreign country they
may mime their needs or demonstrate with objects. Deaf people
can lip read, or use manual sign language or write down what they
want to say. Children who have a language disorder but who are
not autistic communicate in gesture, facial expression and mime.
Children and adults with autism are impaired in using even these
alternative methods of communication.

Before they develop speech, most show their needs by grabbing someone by the hand, pulling them along and putting their
hand on the desired object. It may be years before the children
begin to point and then they usually begin by using their whole
hand rather than pointing with one finger. Only a very few attempt
to mime their needs, and when they do, the movements tend to be
as brief and sketchy as possible.

Simple gestures such as nodding and shaking of the head to
mean yes or no do develop in many of the children but more complex gestures are rare. Some adults do reach the stage of waving

their arms around when speaking, but these movements tend to bear no relation to what is being said.

Attempts are often made to teach manual sign language, such as Makaton, to children and adults with little or no communication. Some will copy signs but never use them spontaneously. Others use them but show the characteristic autistic abnormalities equivalent to those found in oral speech. A few do become able to use this method of communicating effectively. Despite the limitations, teaching manual signs can be helpful for people who have no other way to express their needs.

Young children with autistic disorders have as much trouble understanding non-verbal communication as in using it. As time goes on, however, they begin to have some comprehension of the meaning of clear, simple gestures and expressions. They may then appear to understand more of what is said than they really do because they find clues in people's movements as well as the general context in which communication occurs.

Impairments of Imagination

Children with autistic disorders do not develop pretend play and imaginative activities in the same way as other children. Many never have any kind of pretend play. They handle toys and other objects purely for physical sensations. Some reach the stage of using objects, including miniature toys, for their obvious purposes, such as sweeping with a toy broom or moving trains along a track. A number can perform some quite complex play sequences of this kind but do not act out imaginative stories.

Some of the more-able children do show more evidence of what seems like imagination. They act out a sequence of events that they have invented. This looks convincing at first but prolonged observation shows that the child goes through the same sequence over and over again, without any changes. Most do not involve other children but, if they do, they usually want the others to take part in the same repetitive activity. They do not join in other children's imaginative games. They may reach a stage when they want to take part but do not know how.

Another type of behavior engaged in by some children that appears to be imaginative is the enacting of a character, sometimes copied from television or a book, sometimes an animal or bird or even an inanimate object such as a railway engine. The actions are limited and repetitive, not inventive. The curious feature of this behavior is that the child seems to be living the character or object, rather than pretending.

Many like television and videos but the most popular types of videos and television shows are cartoons, such as *Scooby Doo*, quiz shows with lots of clapping, mechanical noises and flashing lights, science-fiction and films with a lot of action. Soap operas are liked by some because of their familiar characters. Those children who do like to hear stories read to them or recorded on audio-tape want the same ones over and over again, and they know if any word is left out. They do not have an imaginative understanding of the story although they may be able to repeat whole chunks word for word.

The pleasures of creative imagination in childhood are denied to autistic people and so are the rewards in adult life. They have limited or no understanding of other people's emotions, so find it hard to share happiness or sorrow. They are impaired in the ability to share ideas with others and to use past and present experiences to plan for the future. Most of the usual sources of satisfaction are a closed book to people with autism. They find their pleasures in their own special interests.

Repetitive Stereotyped Activities

This aspect of autistic behavior makes most sense if seen as the other side of the coin of impairment of imagination. If the person with autism cannot enjoy the activities that involve flexible, creative thinking, cannot enjoy exchanging ideas with other people, has no understanding of, or interest in, other people and cannot integrate past and present experiences to make plans for the future, the only thing left is the reassurance of repeating those activities that do give some pleasure.

SIMPLE REPETITIVE ACTIVITIES

The simplest forms of these activities involve repetitive sensations. Tasting, smelling, feeling or tapping and scratching different surfaces, listening to mechanical noises, staring at lights or shiny things, twisting and turning hands or objects near the eyes, staring at things from different angles, switching lights on and off, watching things spinning round or self-spinning, are all examples of behavior seen in people with autistic disorders. Sometimes the repetitive activity takes the form of self-biting, head banging, hitting, scratching or other forms of self-injury. More often, behavior of this kind is a response to distress, anger or frustration, but self-injury can be a repetitive habit in someone who has no other way of occupying themselves.

The simple repetitive activities occur mostly in young children. They tend to continue longer in those with the most severe generalized disabilities and may last into adult life.

ELABORATE REPETITIVE ROUTINES

These routines are found especially in children with autism as described by Kanner. There are many variations in the way the pattern is shown.

Some have routines that they invent for themselves, such as tapping on their chair before sitting down, standing up and turning around three times in the course of a meal or carrying out a complex sequence of bodily movements. Placing objects in long lines that must not be disturbed is a familiar feature of autistic behavior. In older children and adults this can take the form of a rigid arrangement of their possessions, which no one must disturb however much dust accumulates.

In other cases the routines derive from an activity initiated usually by the parents, which, having once been done in a certain way, must continue without change. One child always wanted the same route for her daily walk, another insisted that the whole family kept to the same places at the table for every meal. A little boy, in the days before central heating became common, would watch intently as his mother laid the fire and became extremely upset if she did not place the paper, wood and coal in precisely the same pattern every day. Another insisted on a lengthy bedtime routine ending with him lying in the exact center of his bed while his parents arranged the blankets in a special way without any creases. Typically, if the routine is upset there are screams and temper tantrums that can be ended only by starting the routine from the beginning again.

The children may become attached to certain objects and refuse to be parted from them. These may be ordinary toys like dolls or teddy bears, but often they are odd objects such as pieces of string, leaves, tiny squares of photographic negative, little bits of concrete, or pieces of brightly colored plastic. Some children are collectors of such domestic items as empty detergent packets, cans, plastic bottles, or dust pans. They will go to any lengths to add to their store. One little boy, when he realized he had to wait until detergent packets were empty, would throw away the powder from a full packet if it was left in his reach. Another child used to take cans of furniture polish from displays in supermarkets and would even run into people's houses to find such cans if he had the opportunity. He always knew exactly where to look in any house and could run in, grab a can of polish and run out before the house owner realized anything had happened.

Resistance to change can apply to food. Though some children have good appetites from the beginning, others go through a stage in which they refuse to eat more than a few items.

Repetitive acting out of characters and sequences from television series has become fairly common among the children since video recorders have been available. Batman, the Incredible Hulk and the Power Rangers have all been copied in their day. It appears that the children are fascinated by the bizarre, mechanical and repetitive characteristics of the characters they copy. Watching video recordings has had a marked effect on the behavior of children with autistic disorders probably because a video repeats the same events every time it is shown without the slightest variation— the ideal entertainment for the person with autism. Many of the children and adults who are fascinated with certain videos replay the same short sequences so often that the tape breaks.

Music can be the focus of a repetitive routine. Most autistic people are fascinated by music and may play the same tunes on records, cassettes or compact discs over and over again. They may know one conductor's interpretation of a piece and object strongly if they hear another's rendering. Television commercials that combine music and visual stimuli can also become a special interest even if no other programs are watched.

The behaviors described above are most often seen in childhood though they can continue into adult life.

In more able children, especially those with the behavior known as Asperger's syndrome, the elaborate repetitive activities often take the form of fascination with special subjects, such as railway timetables, dinosaurs, the weather, astronomy, science fiction characters and so on ad infinitum. The interest is generally in collecting, memorizing and talking about the facts related to the subjects. For some, there is a special fascination with violence, destruction and death, which can sometimes be combined with high anxiety about these subjects.

The special interest may center around numbers, numerical aspects of objects or complicated calculations. The routines may be complex, as with the young man who could ride a bicycle and insisted on riding to a new town each weekend in strict alphabetical order according to the initial of the name.

This type of complex repetitive behavior often lasts into adult life.

Other Features of Behavior

These behaviors are common but by no means universal and are not crucial for diagnosis.

Movements

STEREOTYPED MOVEMENTS
These movements, often referred to as "stereotypies," occur in most children with autistic disorders and often continue into adult life.

They include finger flicking, flapping arms and hands, jumping up and down, head rolling, rocking while standing up, often springing from back to front foot and making facial grimaces. Many walk on tiptoe, with an odd springy gait.

These movements of hands, limbs and face are most obvious when the child or adult is excited, agitated or angry or is gazing at something that has absorbed their whole attention, such as a spinning object. On the other hand, if they are occupied in some constructive activity, the movements may be minimal or absent.

The reasons for these stereotyped movements are not known for certain. Some could be classified as simple repetitive activities, carried out in order to obtain sensations but others seem to be the result of generalized excitation of the whole body. Body movements with excitement, including arm flapping, are normal in all babies and toddlers. With increasing age there is usually increasing control over such movements but people with autistic disorders appear to remain immature in this respect. They can become tense and distressed if made to suppress their odd movements for long periods of time.

ABNORMALITIES OF GAIT AND POSTURE

Some children with autistic disorders, especially those who fit Kanner's descriptions, are agile climbers and are able to walk along narrow ledges with perfect balance and without fear. Other children, especially those with the behavior described by Asperger, appear clumsy and may be fearful of climbing. Nearly all the children are immature in the way they move. They may not swing their arms appropriately when walking and may walk with head and shoulders bent forward. They may run clumsily with arms outstretched. They may climb or descend stairs standing on each step in turn when they are old enough to alternate their feet. Many of the children have odd postures. They may hold their arms, hands and fingers stretched out or bent at peculiar angles. The abnormalities of gait and posture become more noticeable with increasing age and are most obvious in adolescence and adult life.

Children and adults may be skillful and nimble with their fingers, or they may have poor fine-finger coordination. They tend to do things they want to do with speed and dexterity but have limp or clumsy movements when asked to do things that do not interest them.

Some of the children have difficulty with learning to chew lumpy food, probably because of the difficulties of coordinating the muscles involved in chewing and swallowing. They have to have their food mashed up for them for a longer period of time than normal.

Most children and adults with autism have marked problems with physical education and games. Many of them acquire physical skills they can pursue individually, such as swimming, horseback riding and using trampolines. The problems arise in team sports where they have to coordinate their movements with those of several others, as well as having to remember the rules. The planning and organizing involved in team sports defeats almost all people with autistic disorders, although there is a small minority with skill in one or two team games.

IMITATING MOVEMENTS

Imitation of other people's actions, including facial expressions, should begin in the first year of life. Children with autism typically are delayed in imitating and those most severely affected never do so. It is paradoxical that echoing other people's words is so common, while there are so many problems in copying movements. Parents often find that they have to teach their child with autism to wave, to play baby games and to perform action songs by moving the child's limbs until the action is acquired. All kinds of skills may have to be taught this way because of the lack of any drive to copy others. Some who do begin to imitate, copy other people's actions precisely, but without understanding the meaning. This is known as "echopraxia," a word that is similar to "echolalia" (echoing of speech). Imitation is one of the skills that is basic to developing social behavior, so its impairment is a significant part of the autistic picture.

Responses to Sensory Stimulation

RESPONSES TO SOUNDS

Young children with autistic conditions may be thought to be deaf because they tend not to respond when spoken to and may ignore very loud sounds. They may even fail to blink if someone drops a pile of plates behind them. Parents usually suspect that their child can hear because they notice that he or she responds immediately to some sounds, such as a favorite television commercial jingle, or the sound of chocolate being unwrapped. In his report of 1801, Itard wrote about Victor, the Wild Boy of Aveyron, "Of all his senses the ear appeared the least sensitive. It was found, nevertheless, that the sound of a cracking walnut or other favorite eatable never failed to make him turn round . . . yet this same organ showed itself insensible to the loudest noises and the explosion of firearms."

A child may be fascinated by some sounds such as that made by friction-drive toys or the ringing of a bell. They may find some sounds intensely distressing and will cover their ears and cringe away from, for example, the roar of a motor bike or the barking of a dog or even some comparatively quiet sounds, though they never seem to be sensitive to the noises they make themselves. Ignoring some sounds, fascination with others and distress at yet others may all occur in the same individual.

These odd responses to sounds, especially the over-sensitivity, tend to become less marked with increasing age and may eventually disappear.

RESPONSES TO VISUAL STIMULI

People with autism, especially children, can show the same tendency to be fascinated by, to ignore or to be distressed by visual stimuli as they do to sounds. On the whole, the response of fascination with bright lights is the most common, though some can be overly distressed by, for example, photographic flashes.

When young, some of the children may look at something that moves but lose interest when the movement stops. They seem to recognize people and objects by their general outline rather than by details of their appearance. This suggests that the children may make most use of the peripheral part of the retina that attends to movement and outline, rather than using the central vision for details. Normally, the movement-detecting part of the eye is used mostly in conditions of near darkness, when it is not possible to observe any detail. It is interesting that some of the young children walk, run and even ride a tricycle without seeming to look where they are going and may find their way in the dark quite as easily as in the light. Some young autistic children may not bother to switch on the light if alone in a dark room but can find their own possessions and move around with no difficulty.

These unusual features of response to visual stimuli tend to fade with increasing age.

Responses to Proximal Sensations

This term refers to touch, taste, smell, vibration, pain and temperature, all of which involve direct bodily contact, as distinct from the "distance" senses of hearing and vision. Again, the response can be fascination, distress or indifference. The children seem to explore the world through these senses for much longer than usual. They may touch and lick and smell people as well as objects.

Some children show evident dislike of being touched and will pull away even from gentle, affectionate touches. A few are oversensitive to smells and complain at even faint odors. The feeling of clothing, especially shoes and socks, is disliked by some children. Temple Grandin, a very able adult with autism, wrote in her book, *Emergence: Labeled Autistic,* that when she was a child a starched petticoat felt to her as if she were wearing barbed wire. This is probably why some of the young children remove their clothes, or at least their shoes and socks, whenever they can.

Paradoxically, many of the young children are seemingly indifferent to heat or cold and will want to continue with winter clothes in the summer or run out with little or nothing on in icy weather. One of the most surprising features of autism is the indifference to pain. There are many stories of children with broken bones, dental abscesses, appendicitis or other sources of severe pain who don't complain and behave as if nothing is wrong. They usually do not come for comfort if they hurt themselves. This obliviousness to pain is seen in those with repetitive self-injury.

As with other abnormalities in response to sensory stimuli, these tend to become less marked with age. A child who ignored pain when young may become oversensitive in later childhood and make an enormous fuss about the smallest scratch.

Appetite and Thirst

As already mentioned, insistence on eating only a small range of foods is one form of resistance to change. The child concerned may have a good appetite for the foods they will eat but a few of the children eat very little and, in rare cases, a child will refuse all food. No one knows the reason for this but it does seem as if the child does not recognize the sensation of hunger.

A common feature is excessive drinking of water, fruit juice, tea or other fluids. This can be a major problem if the intake of fluid is so excessive that it leads to vomiting. Thirst does not seem to be the explanation because when they are involved in activities they enjoy the desire to drink seems to be forgotten.

Anxiety and Special Fears

There are some people with autism who appear to have a high level of anxiety most or all of the time. It has been suggested that autistic behavior is the result of severe anxiety from early childhood. This explanation is not convincing because, among many other reasons, most children and adults with autistic disorders are not generally anxious. Their anxiety arises in situations they cannot understand and therefore find confusing and distressing. Furthermore, individuals with autism often do not understand real dangers and are calm when others would be anxious. One family about to go by air to a vacation destination, saw pictures of a plane crash on television on the night before their flight. Their autistic daughter loved watching repairs of broken objects, so her response, said with happy expectation, at the sight of the crashed airplane was the comment, "Man come and mend it." A boy liked the sound of squealing car brakes and would dash in front of cars to make them brake sharply in order to produce this, to him, delightful noise.

It is quite common for the children to develop specific fears of harmless things, such as being bathed, balloons, dogs, riding in buses, even a particular color or shape. These fears can last for years and may create difficulties for the whole family, especially if they are of common everyday objects or events that can hardly be avoided.

Attention and Motivation

Typically, in autistic disorders, attention span is good for activities that interest the child. It may be sustained for a length of time that is surprising, given the age of the child. In contrast, attention for activities or tasks that are outside the range of interests is much shorter and may be fleeting or nonexistent. Given supervision, attention may be held for longer but tends to cease once the guidance is withdrawn. If there are very severe or profound learning difficulties, there may be no special interests and no sustained attention to anything.

The root of the problem in those with good attention when they choose is lack of motivation to engage in anything outside their special interests. For example, there is usually little or no drive to become independent so the child, or even adult, is quite happy to allow a parent or caretaker to dress, wash, even feed them. Left to themselves, children and many adults with autistic disorders are distracted from these self-care tasks by stimuli or activities that fascinate them. As a result, they are so slow in completing the tasks that parents take over when there is a need to hurry. For this reason, parents are often accused of impeding the child's development of independence. The truth is that the demands of ordinary family life make it very difficult to encourage the growth of independence if the children have no interest in doing things for themselves.

Special Skills

Typically, in autistic spectrum disorders there are marked differences in the levels of ability of different kinds of skills on psychological tests. Most often, visuo-spatial skills that do not involve language, like completing jigsaw puzzles, matching shapes and so on, are performed better than skills that need language. A minority do better on verbal tests but these are of the kind that need good rote memory rather than an understanding of abstract ideas or social rules. Since there are exceptions to everything, a few people perform more-or-less equally on all tests.

Perhaps one in ten individuals with autistic spectrum disorders have certain specific skills in which they excel, even in comparison with the normal population. Sometimes the people concerned are of more-or-less average ability in other areas, but there are some individuals who have severe learning difficulties apart from their isolated skills.

The special abilities that have been reported include playing a musical instrument or composing music; performing lengthy numerical calculations such as extracting square roots from huge numbers; identifying the days of the week on which any date fell or will fall in a wide span of years; reading fluently at a very young age though comprehension of the text is poor; memorizing huge quantities of facts about favorite subjects; assembling constructional toys or mechanical or electrical apparatus; working with computers. Some have remarkable drawing ability. The skills depend upon visuo-spatial abilities and/or rote memory. For example, those who draw well remember and reproduce things they have seen. They may be able to rotate mentally something they have seen and draw it from another point of view. It is remarkable that the gifted artists with autistic disorders can draw accurately in perspective from a very young age, unlike other young children who go through many stages before grasping the rules of perspective. Sometimes they will draw only in one medium such as with a blue ball-point pen, or on steam on a window. With crayons, for example, their drawings might be childish. These skills tend to become a focus for the repetitive routines. Thus the drawings are of the same subjects, the music is played repetitively, the calendar calculators want to be fed dates all the time.

Some of those with special skills at some time in childhood or adult life cease using them. The reason for this is unknown, nor is it clear whether the skills are lost or just no longer used. They are rarely taken up again despite any amount of encouragement. One child stopped her remarkable drawings when her speech developed but there is no general evidence that speech and visuo-spatial skills are incompatible.

Inappropriate Behavior

Inappropriate, difficult behavior is frequent in children with autistic disorders. The causes include confusion and fear of unfamiliar situations; interference with repetitive routines; failure to understand social rules; inappropriate attempts to control events; oversensitivity to sensory input from loud sounds, bright lights, crowds of people; pursuit of preferred activities without any ability to consider the consequences.

In the family home, the children can be restless, destructive, noisy, aggressive if frustrated and given to running away if the opportunity occurs. They may sleep very little and disturb the family when awake. Their demands and their routines may eventually take priority over all the family's other needs because of the severity of the temper tantrums if the child is thwarted in any way.

Often, behavior in public is as difficult as it is at home. The children who are given to screaming are not inhibited by being in a public place and will scream as loud and long in the street as at home. They may take things off store counters, run round the aisles of supermarkets, lie on the floor in a temper tantrum or run into the street regardless of traffic. The young children have no idea that it is not appropriate to take off one's clothes in public and may happily disrobe to sit in an inviting puddle of rain water, if so inclined. They may touch the hair, clothing, wristwatch or other possessions of strangers, ignoring any protests. The problems may be so severe that the parents cannot take the child with them when they shop, and vacations away from home are impossible.

The children who have good language may be more amenable but they can cause small social crises. They do not understand that some things are better left unsaid. They may talk about topics that are not mentioned in polite society. Innocently, they make inappropriate remarks. All young children are liable to be tactless but the tendency is more marked and goes on to a much later age in children who are autistic. One girl of twelve, who spoke very well, on seeing an unusually short woman, said, in her loud, clear voice, "Mommy, look at that dear little lady." A child, looking at a newborn infant, commented to the proud mother, "What an awful face." Most people with autism, even those with good speech, never tell lies. They do not understand why it should ever be necessary to avoid the truth and, in any case, lack the skill with language and ideas needed to invent lies. If they do reach the stage of telling lies this is done without any subtlety and is easily detected. Some tell fantastic stories about their favorite themes but these are not motivated by the desire to deceive. The sources of such stories are usually easily recognized and tend to be based on television, books, or films.

The social naivete can lead to inappropriately friendly approaches to strangers. Parents of the more-able adolescents worry about the possible dangers in this behavior and feel they have to restrict their child's freedom on this account.

Just like young normal children, children with autistic disorders tend to pick up bad language and terms of abuse. Unlike normal children they are unaware of the need for discretion and may use swear words on most unsuitable occasions.

People outside the family may blame the parents for "spoiling" their child but no one who has not had direct experience can know what it is like to live with an autistic child. Children with autistic conditions are totally egocentric, not because of deliberate selfishness but because they do not understand that others have thoughts or feelings. They lack any desire to please and most have no anxiety about parental displeasure. The usual ways of interacting with children and teaching them social rules do not apply in this situation. However, there are ways of helping to make behavior more appropriate, as will be discussed in Chapter 11.

Epileptic Seizures

Seizures cannot, strictly speaking, be classified as "behavior" but they are included in this description because they are a commonly occurring part of the clinical picture.

Among the children who have learning difficulties as well as autistic disorders, about one quarter to one third, have had at least one epileptic seizure by the time they reach adult life. Seizures can occur in those of average or higher levels of ability but are much less common. They may begin in infancy, childhood, adolescence, or even in adult life. In some, the seizures occur only with a fever. Some teenagers may have one or two and then no more. Other children or adolescents have recurrent seizures for many years or all their lives. Any type of seizure may be seen among those with autistic disorders.

Changes with Growing Up

Autistic behavior tends to be most obvious to the parents and most typical in the years from two to five. The exception to this occurs among the most-able children with little or no delay in language development. Their parents may attribute their lack of interest in other children and their determination to go their own way as evidence of a strong character and high intelligence. Problems in this group typically become recognized when they start school, refuse to fit into the classroom or playground activities and appear indifferent to any rewards or sanctions.

In children who have shown marked autistic behavior in their early years, changes often occur around five to six years. In some children, the autistic behavior becomes much less obvious. There are children who seem to lose all the typical abnormalities apart from a few subtle signs in their social relationships. For some, the clinical picture becomes that of a pure developmental language disorder, with few if any autistic features. In the majority of children, the autistic behavior remains clearly present although, in most, varying degrees of improvement in skills and behavior occur.

For all children, adolescence is another time of change. Some go through this stage of life without any special problems and may even improve markedly. In others, there is a return of the temper tantrums, aggression or other inappropriate behavior seen in the early years.

By adult life, the ways in which autistic behavior is manifested become even more varied. The most disabled are completely dependent on others and still show the autistic characteristics seen in childhood. At the other end of the scale, the most able are living and working independently and some are married with children. The problems that remain are the subtle impairments of social interaction and communication, though some compensate for these by studying and following the example of other people. In some people, the picture is complicated by a psychiatric illness (see Chapter 14).

Follow-up studies have shown that the most important factor in deciding the amount of intellectual progress is the overall level of ability, which can be measured in childhood by psychological tests of language and visuo-spatial skills, as long as these are given by people with skill and experience. These are reliable guides if the child is tested after five years of age. The education and care experienced during childhood can affect behavior and can help the child to develop potential skills more quickly, but do not seem to make a significant difference in the final level. In addition to these factors, the individuals most likely to become independent are those with an equable temperament, who have special skills and interests that can be used for paid employment and who have a strong desire to succeed in the world.

CHAPTER 4

How Many Children Have Autistic Disorders?

Prevalence

All the studies concerning the numbers of people with autistic disorders have counted children and adolescents but, so far, have not included adults. The studies have been of prevalence—that is, the number of cases in the specified age range living in the specified geographical area at the time the count was made. The term incidence is sometimes used but this should properly refer only to the number of new cases in a specified time. For autistic disorders, this might be the number of new cases in one year. This would be very difficult to count because of the impossibility at present of making a diagnosis at birth. However, a recent study of 18-month-old children has given some indication of incidence, and rough calculations of incidence can be made from the estimates of prevalence.

A number of studies have investigated the prevalence of typical autism. This type of study counts the numbers of people in a defined geographical area who fit the criteria of the research. A review of 16 such studies, from the U.S., Canada, Britain, Scandinavia, France and Japan, that published their findings between 1966 and 1991, found that prevalence rates varied from 2 to 16 cases per 10,000 children. As noted in the Introduction, the first-ever prevalence study, by Victor Lotter, that counted children with Kanner's criteria—that is, severe lack of affective contact (social aloofness) and insistence on elaborate repetitive routines—found a rate of 4.5 per 10,000 children. Other studies in the U.K. and Denmark, carried out in the 1960s and '70s, that strictly applied Kanner's criteria, also found four to five affected children in every 10,000. Studies using the wider definitions of "typical" autism as given in the DSM or ICD systems mostly found the higher rates.

The study in Camberwell Judith Gould and I carried out in the 1970s (mentioned in the Introduction) used the broadest definition of autistic spectrum disorders—that is, all those with the triad of impairments. We included children who had the triad even if they had other conditions as well. We screened all children in the borough born between 1956 and 1970 who had special needs. Almost all of these had mild, moderate or severe learning difficulties (IQ under 70). We concentrated on them because early studies of Kanner's autism had shown that most had some degree of difficulty with learning. We found about 20 in every 10,000 children had the triad, including those with Kanner's autism. We examined the children and made the diagnoses. Very few had previously been recognized as autistic. In 1986, Gillberg and his colleagues in Gothenburg, Sweden, in a study of children with learning disabilities, reported similar rates.

Later, the same group of workers in Sweden examined children aged 7 to 16 years (born 1975 to 1983) in mainstream schools (with IQ 70 or above). They found 36 per 10,000 fitted Asperger's syndrome and another 35 per 10,000 who had social impairment but did not fit perfectly either Kanner's or Asperger's syndromes. Adding together the rates from the two studies gives a grand total for all autistic spectrum disorders of 91 per 10,000 or nearly one in 100. It must be emphasized that these numbers included, in Camberwell, children with profound learning disabilities and, in Gothenburg, children with high levels of ability and only subtle symptoms. These studies have been criticized because they were based on small populations but they had the advantage of being very thorough.

More recent population studies in the U.K. and Sweden have found rates around 40 to 50 or more per 10,000. The California Health and Human Services Agency has examined the numbers of people diagnosed as having autistic spectrum disorders entering the California Developmental Services system each year from 1987 on and has found a substantial rise. However, it is not yet possible to calculate the true annual population rates accurately from this information.

Are the Numbers Increasing?

As a result of recent publications on prevalence, this question is frequently asked by professionals working with children. Many feel sure that they are seeing more children with autistic disorders than they did in the past.

There are three possible reasons for the reported rise in prevalence. First, there has been a marked widening of the definition of autism and autistic spectrum disorders. Even the definition of typical autism (called "autistic disorder" in the DSM-IV classification) is much broader than the narrow criteria of aloofness and elaborate repetitive routines demanded by Leo Kanner for his classic autism. The spread of knowledge of Asperger's work has affected diagnostic theory and practice. Second, there has been a steadily growing interest in autistic disorders of all kinds among both professionals and parents. A child is much more likely to be recognized as having autism now than 10 to 15 years ago. Third, there may be a real increase. The true answer may be that one, or two, or even all three of these factors are present. In this context it is worth pointing out that the combined Camberwell and Gothenburg studies of children born between 1956 and 1983 gave a higher rate for all autistic spectrum disorders than any of the other studies, even the most recent ones. This suggests that changing definitions and increasing awareness may, on their own, account for the reported increase in rates.

It is reasonable to ask, if the rate has always been higher than supposed, where are the adults with autistic disorders who were not diagnosed as children? In the first decades of the 20th century, many young children with autistic behavior were placed in the old institutions. Now that there has been a change to community rather than institutional care, and a complete change in attitude to the needs of people with disabilities, the children are being seen by community pediatricians and other professionals instead of being institutionalized. In my own experience of the now-defunct institutions for adults with learning disabilities, about one-third of the residents had autistic spectrum disorders. These were diagnosed by my colleagues and me as part of our research—in most cases the diagnoses had not been made before we saw the people concerned.

The definitive evidence needed to prove or disprove a real rise in prevalence of autistic spectrum disorders is not available. If it were possible to do a series of studies from now on, they might show that numbers are still rising, or falling, or staying the same, or that they fluctuate from time to time or place to place—but there is no way of finding out what has happened in the past.

If there has been a marked rise, the reasons are unknown. Explanations, such as the effects of pollution, additives in the diet, or the evils of the urban environment, have all been suggested, but there is no evidence for any of these theories. At the time of this writing, there is great concern that the triple measles, mumps and rubella (MMR) vaccine can cause autism. There is no solid evidence for this theory either. It is discussed in more detail in Chapter 6.

Age of Onset

Kanner at first believed that his syndrome was always present from birth, so he named it "early infantile autism." Later he observed the same syndrome in children who appeared to have had a year or two of normal development before becoming autistic. As previously noted, the ICD-10 and DSM-IV criteria specify onset before three years of age for typical autism. Onset of the behavioral pattern after this age is referred to in these systems as "atypical autism."

There can be problems in sorting out the age at which autistic behavior first appeared. Parents may not realize that their child's behavior is unusual until the second or third year. At this time they may begin to worry because their child is slow in talking and shows intense resistance to change. Careful questioning usually shows that problems were present from birth or early infancy (see Chapter 3) but, occasionally, there does seem to have been a period of normal development followed by a real change to autistic behavior. This is typically in the second or third year but may be later.

Sometimes this onset follows a fever, perhaps due to encephalitis (a virus infection of the brain) or some kind of trauma, but there may be no apparent reason. It can follow an event such as a house move or birth of a sibling. Enough is now known about the essentially physical causes of autistic disorders to suggest that such psychological stresses affect children who were vulnerable and would have developed autistic behavior in any case.

The latest DSM and ICD criteria for Asperger's syndrome specify normal development in speech and adaptive skills before three years (see Chapter 2) but this conflicts with diagnoses based on the behavior pattern alone. Specifying ages of onset as essential criteria for diagnosis causes all sorts of problems. All the evidence is based on parents' memories of the early years, unless the child is seen and assessed while very young. Parents can usually describe behavior but tend to be less accurate in dating events. If the parents are not available when trying to assess someone seen for the first time as an adult, diagnosis is theoretically impossible. It is better to diagnose based on the overall pattern as revealed in the history rather than on an arbitrary cut-off point based on age.

Number of Boys Compared with Girls

Boys are affected more often than girls. Kanner found four times as many boys among children with his autistic syndrome. Asperger at first thought that girls were never affected with his syndrome but later changed his mind. The Swedish study of Asperger's syndrome in mainstream schools found a ratio of four boys to one girl.

There is some evidence that, although girls have autistic disorders less often than boys, when they are affected they are likely to be more severely disabled. The higher prevalence among boys is most obvious with those of high ability and the difference decreases when the level of overall intelligence is lower. There are some very able women with autistic disorders but far fewer than men. The study in Sweden also identified a group who had some but not all of the criteria for Asperger's syndrome. When these cases were included the ratio changed to 2.3 boys to 1 girl, suggesting that autistic disorders may be more difficult to recognize in girls.

As with so many aspects of autistic disorders, the reasons for this sex difference is unknown. Perhaps the social instincts of girls are stronger than those of boys so it takes more severe damage to impair them in a girl. Asperger was brave enough to suggest that his syndrome was the extreme end of the continuum of the normal male personality. Solving this question may have relevance to many issues of gender differences.

Parents' Occupations

Almost all the autistic children seen by Kanner had fathers who were of higher intelligence and educational level than average and most had professional occupations. Kanner believed that this was a special feature of autism. Many of the earlier studies of children with Kanner's autism seen at various centers found the same tendency in the parents' occupations, though never to the marked extent described by Kanner. Any sample based on a clinic may be biased by special selection factors. It is probable that parents with professional qualifications were more likely to have heard of Kanner's work and to have had the determination and the means to attend his clinic.

In order to examine this question properly, it is necessary to look at the results of studies that identified all children with autism in a specified area, regardless of whether they had been referred to a special clinic. Out of the 16 prevalence studies published between 1966 and 1991 (mentioned above), nine gave information on parents' occupations. In only two of these was any bias toward higher economic and educational class reported and in neither was it anywhere near as large as Kanner had found. It is no longer assumed that autistic disorders occur more often in families of higher occupational status, though studies specifically concerned with the most able group, especially those who have the behavior pattern described by Asperger, have not yet been carried out.

CHAPTER 5

Conditions Associated with Autistic Spectrum Disorders

Autistic disorders are a result of problems with particular aspects of development, so many of the typical features of behavior are due to extreme immaturity. They appear peculiar only because they are discrepant with the age of the individual and when compared with skill levels in other areas.

Everything that a child with an autistic disorder does, other children may do at some time or other during their development. Young children who are developing normally can flap their arms with excitement, jump and run around in circles while playing. The age when children begin to talk varies. Children have temper tantrums; they may hold on to a piece of cloth or a teddy bear and weep when it is lost; specific fears are common and so are food fads. With growing independence, especially in the second year, young children can be very uncooperative and inclined to ignore instructions and to say no to every suggestion.

The difference is that in a child whose social development is progressing along normal lines, these things happen in passing phases, whereas they continue for years on end in children with autistic disorders. When children who are not autistic reach the appropriate stage of development, normally in the second year, they begin to have imaginative play and varied activities, whereas children with autistic disorders are limited and repetitive in the things they do. Most important of all, children who are not autistic have a strong drive to take part in social interaction, communication and play, especially with their age peers.

When making a diagnosis and considering whether developmental disorders other than autism are present, it is important to be aware that autistic spectrum disorders can occur together with any other disability, physical or psychological. If the triad of impairments of social interaction, communication, and imagination is present, then an autistic disorder should be diagnosed regardless of any other coexisting condition. The triad cannot be explained away by another disability. The question must always be "Does this child have an autistic disorder *and* (not or) some other condition?" The importance of recognizing the autistic disorder is the major factor in determining what type of care and education are needed by the child, no matter what other condition might exist.

Generalized Learning Difficulties

Learning difficulties and autistic disorders often but by no means always occur together. In autistic disorders specific aspects of the skills needed for adapting to social life are always impaired. However, other abilities may or may not be affected, at least as far as obtaining scores on psychological tests of intelligence is concerned. Autistic disorders can be found at any level of ability, from profoundly disabled up to average or higher abilities.

Considering the whole range of autistic disorders, including the type described by Asperger, about one third have learning difficulties, the majority of these being severely or profoundly learning disabled. Most of those in the Asperger group have test scores in the low-average range or better. Of those with autism like that described by Kanner, about one third have severe to moderate learning difficulties, one-third have mild difficulties and one-third are in the low-average or better range. Conversely, 50 to 60 percent of all children with severe or profound learning difficulties also have the triad of impairments but the proportion is very much lower, at around 0.2 to 0.4 percent, among those with mild learning difficulties or average and above ability.

Among children or adults with severe learning difficulties, there are some who function at such a low level that they have not reached the stages of development at which language and pretend play emerge. Their activities tend to be repetitive and many have stereotyped movements. Diagnosis has to be based on social responsiveness as shown in facial expression, eye contact and bodily movements. At this level, autistic disorder is just one of many problems. However, recognizing that an autistic disorder is present helps parents and other caretakers to understand that the lack of social responsiveness is not related to any fault in the love and care being given. They can also be aware of the types of stimuli, such as loud sounds, that might cause distress and the activities, such as a sensory room, that might be enjoyed.

Is generalized learning disability part of the autistic disorder or is it due to additional brain dysfunction, perhaps produced by the same original cause as the autism but with a different site for the brain pathology? The answer to this question is not yet known. It is most likely that both situations can occur. Autistic disorders adversely affect the ability to learn from social interaction and to make sense out of experiences and this must reduce the capacity to learn and make use of information. The children and adults who score well on tests mostly do so on the strength of their good rote memories and their visuo-spatial not their verbal reasoning abilities. On the other hand, some of the medical conditions associated with autism do give rise to pathological changes in various parts of the brain of which some may be relevant to autistic disorders and others to learning difficulties.

Whatever the causes of the association between autistic disorders and generalized learning difficulties, it is important to consider both separately when making a diagnosis. The presence of one does not explain away the presence of the other.

Rett's Syndrome

This is a very rare syndrome that so far has been reported only in girls. After a few months of apparently normal development, the child gradually loses the ability to use her hands to hold and manipulate objects. Repetitive movements of the hands occur, mainly

hand wringing or rubbing or tapping both hands together. Head
growth slows or stops. Walking is very poor and the child may
sooner or later have to use a wheelchair. Curvature of the spine may
develop. Overbreathing, air-swallowing and teeth-grinding are common. With the onset of these problems, the child often shows signs
of anxiety and becomes socially cut off. There is very severe learning
disability, little or no language development and no pretend play.
The picture at this stage is like that of an autistic disorder in a severely disabled child. It is interesting that over a varying length of
time the children often lose the autistic social impairment and become responsive to social approaches, though retaining all the other
features of the autistic syndrome. Rett's Syndrome is associated
with an abnormality of a gene on the X chromosome.

Fragile X Syndrome

This is an inherited condition due to an abnormality of the X chromosome. It is more common and more marked in males. Certain
physical abnormalities, including large ears and a long face, occur
in differing degrees of severity. Learning difficulties of varying levels,
motor stereotypes, over-sensitivity to sound and to touch, repetitive routines and abnormalities of speech are part of the usual picture. Hyperactivity and poor attention span may be seen in the
children. The social behavior is of particular interest. Eye contact is
usually avoided and the affected individuals tend to keep a physical distance from other people. However, their social difficulties appear to arise from shyness, anxiety and the dislike of being touched
rather than from social aloofness and indifference. The quality is
different from that in an autistic condition. In a few cases, the autistic type of social impairment occurs. These account for only a small
proportion of all people with autistic disorders but chromosome
examination for Fragile X is now a standard part of the investigation of autistic behavior.

Landau-Kleffner Syndrome

This very rare disorder occurs in children, usually between three
and seven years of age, whose development was previously normal,

although some have delay in language development. The first signs may be behavioral changes or problems affecting language. Many have autistic-like features such as poor eye contact, repetitive routines and resistance to change. The pattern of the encephalogram (EEG) is typically abnormal but this may be detected only if special techniques of recording are used. There may be seizures but these do not always occur. Steroid drugs offer marked improvements in behavior. Anti-epileptic drugs are also used. A form of brain surgery has been developed to treat this condition and is reported to give good results in some children.

Other Neurological Conditions

Many physical conditions known to affect the brain can be associated with autistic disorders or aspects of autistic behavior. Certain conditions that are congenital or that occur in the first year or two of life are likely to be associated with autistic disorders as well as learning difficulties and, often, epilepsy. The major ones are tuberose sclerosis, a genetic condition giving patches of abnormal tissue in the brain, skin and other organs; untreated phenylketonuria, another genetic condition causing a biochemical abnormality that can be treated with a special diet if diagnosed in infancy; some viral and other infections in the mother during pregnancy, particularly rubella; infantile spasms, a rare and severe form of epilepsy occurring in the first year of life. Encephalitis from various kinds of viral infections, especially if it occurs in the early years of life, can also give rise to an autistic disorder. There are various other conditions associated with learning difficulties and epilepsy in which autistic disorders occasionally occur.

A number of other congenital conditions, some known to be genetic while in others the cause is not yet known, often have, in addition to the physical abnormalities, one or more features of behavior that occur in autistic disorders but not the whole picture. Fragile X has already been mentioned. Two other examples are Williams syndrome, also known as infantile hypercalcemia, in which repetitive speech and questioning and naive, inappropriate social approaches are common, and Cornelia de Lange syndrome, in which self-injury can be a severe problem. Tourette's syndrome is a neurological disorder in which the symptoms include grunting and twitching, obsessions, uttering of obscenities, attention deficits and over-activity. In any of these conditions, an autistic disorder in its full form can occasionally occur.

Diagnosis of all these conditions depends upon recognition of the physical signs and the history and observation of the behavior pattern. Autistic behavior has to be taken into account and properly managed even if it is associated with a known physical condition.

Severe Hearing Impairments

Children who are born with severe hearing impairments have many problems in learning to understand and use spoken language. They may be difficult in their behavior and have some features of behavior seen in autistic children when they are young. However, if they are not autistic as well as hearing-impaired, they form social attachments and are able to use gestures, facial expression, miming and eventually a sign language to communicate and they develop pretend play.

Autistic disorders can occur together with any degree of deafness in which case the dual diagnosis must be made. It is important to make sure that children with autistic behavior are not also deaf. Testing is often a difficult problem, but the parents' observations of their child's behavior at home can be helpful in making a decision.

Severe Visual Impairments

Some children with severe congenital visual impairments who seem to be developing normally at birth begin to show autistic behavior in their second or third year of life. Some who are born with a combination of severe visual and hearing impairments have autistic behavior, especially those affected by maternal rubella. The onset of autistic behavior in these children, whether from birth or in the second or third year, seems likely to be due to associated brain damage rather than the sensory impairments alone.

Some people with congenital visual impairments have stereo-typed movements, possibly to compensate for the lack of visual stimulation, but do not have any other features of autistic behavior.

Developmental Language Disorders

Children with these difficulties have problems with spoken language. Those with "receptive" problems have difficulty in understanding words and therefore in learning to speak. Those with "expressive" problems can understand reasonably well but have difficulty in producing words for themselves. Difficulties with articulation can occur without receptive or expressive disorders. Some children have mixtures of all these aspects of language disorder.

The children with receptive language disorders, especially when young, tend to ignore sounds and to be socially withdrawn. However, if they have the disorder in pure form, they use gestures, eye pointing, facial expression and miming to communicate and can learn a formal sign language. If they learn to read and write they can communicate through writing. They do relate to others and develop imaginative play even if they tend to be developmentally immature. In pure form, receptive language disorders are comparatively rare. Difficulties in language comprehension are, of course, very common in autistic disorders. When children are young, receptive difficulties may be ascribed to a pure language disorder even though other aspects of the triad of impairments are present. This is not helpful for the child or the family because it delays the provision of the right education and advice and help for the parents. The correct diagnosis must be made on a full history and current picture of behavior, not on language tests alone. There are some children on the borderline between autism and receptive language disorder in whom diagnosis is difficult. The important point is to assess the precise nature of the impairments in each individual child and to tailor the educational and behavior management programs to their specific needs.

Children with pure expressive language disorders can understand speech. They can use non-spoken methods of communication, are usually sociable, though immature, and have pretend play. Expressive problems may be associated with poor motor coordination. They can also occur together with autistic disorders.

Semantic-Pragmatic Disorder

The idea of the existence of this syndrome was first put forward only a few years ago. It is described as a condition in which speech production is fluent and grammatically correct but there is a serious deficit in the understanding of speech. There is much repetition and often immediate and delayed echolalia. The children have good memories and may read precociously but with poor understanding. The pragmatic aspect of language is its use in social conversation and its relevance to situations. This is markedly impaired in the syndrome. Some have special interests and repetitive routines. As pointed out by Sarah Lister Brook and Dermot Bowler, who compared the published studies on this subject, this is a description of the "active but odd" group among the autistic disorders, including those who can be diagnosed as having Asperger's syndrome. Some professional workers who are specialists in linguistics or language therapy insist that the semantic-pragmatic disorder can exist separately from the autistic spectrum. This is usually because they concentrate on language without examining the whole pattern of behavior and the development from infancy of children given this diagnosis. Most people in the field of autistic disorders do not consider that there is any value in separating semantic-pragmatic disorder from the autistic spectrum. The disadvantage of doing so is the failure to recognize the child's whole pattern of disabilities and therefore a failure to address all their needs. It is also most misleading for the parents.

Disorders of Attention, Motor Coordination and Perception

Each of these developmental disorders can occur on its own or in combination. They can be associated with language disorders, hyperactivity or under-activity. The perceptual problems include muddling letters in words and letter and word reversals and are associated with difficulties in learning to read, write and spell. Insistence on following routines and resistance to change are common. Christopher Gillberg and his colleagues in Sweden have found that among children who have a combination of the disorders of attention, motor coordination and perception, referred to as the DAMP syndrome, there are a number who have diagnosable autistic disorders, especially in the form described by Asperger. As with all developmental disorders, it is important to take a detailed history and to identify each element that may be present and its level of severity, rather than deciding that one of the conditions explains all the other features.

Elective Mutism

A small number of children talk in one situation (for example, at home) but remain silent elsewhere (for example, at school). Shyness and reluctance to speak in strange situations is fairly common in toddlers when first beginning to speak, but if it goes on until school age it is a cause for concern.

"Elective mutism," as this behavior is called, can be associated with a variety of speech and behavior problems including autistic disorders. The aim of diagnosis is to find the reason for the behavior. This, as always, requires a full history from infancy and details of the child's whole pattern of behavior in different settings, the way language is used when the child does speak and whether the child uses non-spoken methods of communication. The term "elective mutism" is a name for a specific type of behavior, not a diagnosis in itself, so it does not explain away autistic behavior if it is present.

Psychiatric Conditions

Any type of psychiatric condition can complicate autistic disorders, especially in adolescence and early adult life (see Chapter 15). Difficulties of diagnosis and treatment frequently arise because the psychiatrist, in addition to knowledge of adult psychiatric illness, also has to be aware of autistic spectrum disorders as they appear in adolescents and adults, especially those who are more able. Diagnostic errors are of three types, any of which can lead to inappropriate recommendations for treatment, services and longer-term care.

The first type of error is mistaking an uncomplicated autistic disorder for a psychiatric illness. Adults of borderline, average or high ability with undiagnosed autistic disorders have been wrongly labeled as suffering from any and every psychiatric condition. Among the most common misdiagnoses are obsessive compulsive disorder, depression and schizophrenia. It is necessary to take a developmental history from a parent covering all the relevant details in order to make the correct diagnosis.

Very rarely, psychiatric conditions usually seen in adolescence or adult life, including schizophrenia, can occur in childhood and lead to strange behavior. These have to be differentiated from autistic disorders on the history and observation of behavior. Childhood schizophrenia is extremely rare and has not been reported as beginning before the age of seven. Confusion over diagnosis is most likely with the type of child with an autistic disorder who makes active but odd social approaches and who has a lot of repetitive speech and pseudo-pretend play. The diagnosis of schizophrenia should be made only if the delusions and hallucinations characteristic of that condition are reported by the child, which means that it can be diagnosed only if the child has enough speech.

The diagnosis of "schizoid personality disorder" has caused some confusion. The term "personality disorder" is used to cover various patterns of behavior that are markedly different from the usual culturally accepted range and are consistent and typical of the individual concerned but are not explained by psychiatric illness. The problem is that the factors underlying personality, whether normal or deviant, are still unknown. In the case of "schizoid personality" the descriptions that have been written of people with this label have certainly included some who had autistic spectrum disorders, especially of the kind described by Asperger. The ICD-10 criteria for schizoid personality disorder include such items as emotional detachment, limited capacity to display warmth to others, consistent choice of solitary activities and no close friends, all of which occur in autistic disorders.

An investigation by Digby Tantam of adults who fit the diagnostic criteria for "schizoid personality" showed that many had the
developmental history diagnostic of autistic spectrum disorders.
Some workers have used the label "schizoid personality" for young
adults who behaved exactly like Asperger described from early
childhood onward. Obviously what has happened is that psychiatrists who work with children and those who work only with adults
have each seen the same kinds of people but at different stages of
their lives and have given the same people different labels. The
range of clinical pictures covered by the term "schizoid personality disorder" is not identical with autistic spectrum disorders in
more-able people but there is much overlap. When there is a choice,
which label is best? The answer is to choose the one that is most
helpful for the person concerned. The label "personality disorder"
is vague and general and has no useful implications. The term
"schizoid personality disorder" suggests a link with schizophrenia
but there is no evidence that people with autistic conditions are
any more likely than anyone else to develop schizophrenia in adult
life. Saying that someone has a "schizoid personality" gives no guidance on treatment or the kinds of help and services they require.
In contrast, classification as autistic spectrum disorder, which is
recognized as a developmental disorder, leads to an investigation
of precisely which aspects of development are affected and then to
consideration of what can be done to alleviate the problems. This
approach has had major practical implications for ways of helping
people with autistic spectrum disorders, so this diagnostic classification is the one to be recommended.

The second type of error is missing a psychiatric illness com-
plicating an autistic disorder. This is easy to do because of the difficulty of obtaining a full and coherent history of symptoms from
the person with an autistic disorder. Information from parents or
other caregivers is essential, especially concerning any recent
changes from the usual pattern of behavior.

The third type of error is diagnosing a psychiatric illness but
failing to recognize the presence of an underlying autistic disorder.
This can happen when there is good evidence of a psychiatric illness

but no parent has been asked for a relevant developmental history. It helps if the psychiatrist who diagnoses and treats the psychiatric illness has some experience with adults with autistic disorders and is alert for oddities of social interaction and communication.

Effects of Deprivation

Babies and young children who are seriously deprived of stimulating experiences, especially close contact and communication with a caring person, are held back in social, language and intellectual development. They may be so withdrawn and unresponsive that they give the impression of being autistic. Careful observation of the full behavior pattern shows the differences, but the most important point for diagnosis is the effect of providing the child with better care and wider experiences. Within a few weeks or even days of being given such care, the deprived child begins to make strides in development in all areas. The progress of a child with an autistic disorder, on the other hand, is painfully slow and the basic handicaps remain, even after years of loving care and patient teaching.

Clarke and Clarke, in their book *Early Experience: Myths and Evidence*, give some most interesting examples of deprived children who were eventually rescued. They discuss the unsolved question as to how long severe deprivation has to continue before the effects on the child become irreversible. Difficulties in diagnosis arise if a child who has severe learning difficulties or an autistic disorder also happens to be deprived in the early years. The temptation is to explain the handicaps as resulting from the poor environment, but a careful consideration of all the evidence shows the inappropriateness of this type of explanation.

At this time, studies are being carried out on children who suffered severe physical and emotional deprivation in Romanian orphanages and who were later adopted by families in other countries. These studies may help shed light on the reasons for the wide variations in the degree to which different children recover from deprivation. Clarke and Clarke, in their second book *Early Experience and the Life Path*, discuss the preliminary findings of the work in this field.

CHAPTER 6

What Causes Autistic Spectrum Disorders?

When the first edition of this book was written in 1971 there were still many professionals who believed the theories that autism was caused by the way parents brought up their children. At that time it was necessary to review in detail the arguments for and against these ideas. There was never any scientific evidence to support this view. As soon as properly controlled studies were carried out it became evident that such theories were wrong. Now, no one with a sound knowledge of research in the field holds such beliefs because the evidence for a physical cause leading to a disorder of development is so strong. The frequency of epilepsy and of generalized learning difficulties is a clinical indicator of brain dysfunction, quite apart from findings from special techniques of examination. The search is on for the nature of the physical cause or, more likely, causes.

Research into causation is being pursued at three different but interrelated levels—the original causes; the site and nature of the pathology in the brain produced by the original causes and the impairments of psychological function produced by the brain pathology; and how these lead to the observable abnormalities of behavior. It is a scientific version of the House that Jack Built.

Original Causes

Associated Medical Conditions

Studies have shown that a variety of specific medical conditions liable to produce brain pathology can be associated with autistic disorders. Some of these have been mentioned in Chapter 5. There are differing opinions among research workers as to the proportion of children whose typical autism appears to originate from an identifiable medical condition. The best estimates come from epidemiological studies where all eligible children are seen and examined because, if a child has, for instance, tuberose sclerosis, associated autism may not be recognized and no referral made to a specialist clinic. Figures from the epidemiological studies of typical autism vary because of differences in selection criteria but it appears that about one-quarter have an identifiable medical condition that probably caused the autism. Such conditions are most likely to be found among those with severe or profound generalized learning difficulties, though they can occur in individuals of any level of ability.

Perinatal Problems

Problems during the birth process tend to be significantly more common than average among children with autistic disorders. In the past it was thought that these might be the cause of some congenital disabilities, including autism. However, most researchers now consider some difficult births are related to pre-existing abnormalities in the child. It appears that the baby has to contribute to the birth process, and prenatal abnormalities in development can cause difficulties. This is of particular interest because a considerable amount of evidence now shows that, in addition to the genetic medical conditions associated with autistic behavior, such as tuberose sclerosis, genetic factors are important in many cases of autistic disorders.

Genetics

Studies of twins and of family histories have shown positive correlations. The patterns in families indicate that the cause is not simply a single dominant or recessive gene. The mechanism must be complex and certainly involves several genes in combination. Research teams in different countries are currently engaged in attempts to locate the chromosomes and genes responsible for the pathology of autistic disorders, particularly in autism of the type described by Kanner, though it is already clear that more than one type of autistic disorder as well as other developmental delays or disabilities can occur within one extended family. A study by Patrick Bolton and his colleagues published in 1994 suggested that, among siblings of children with typical autism, nearly three percent also had typical autism and the same number had other pervasive developmental disorders (autistic spectrum disorders). The diagnoses were based on the criteria from the international classification system (ICD-10). The researchers also looked for more subtle impairments of communication and social interaction and repetitive patterns of behavior that were insufficient to justify a diagnosis of an autistic spectrum disorder. They found that 20 percent of the siblings had one or more of these impairments, albeit in very subtle form. The children were compared with an age- and sex-matched group of children with Down's syndrome who did not have autism. The Down's syndrome children had no siblings with autistic disorders and only three percent had siblings with subtle impairments. It appears that, unless the siblings of Down's syndrome children are particularly unlikely to have autistic-type impairments, the siblings of children with typical autism are much more likely to have autism or autistic-like traits than the general population. Recent work suggests that genes on chromosome 7 may be implicated, but which genes are crucial and how they affect development is still not known.

Although the evidence gathered from twin and family studies for the importance of genetics in autistic disorders is strong, it is also clear that other factors must be involved. For example, identical twins can show markedly different types of autistic disorders and may have disabilities with very different levels of severity, which may result from pre- or postnatal influences.

Disorders of Feeding and Bowel Function

A theme that runs through a number of different theories about the nature of autistic disorders is the occurrence of abnormalities of feeding and bowel function in the children and adults with these conditions. Feeding problems in infancy are common. In childhood, strange types of food fads are often seen, as described in the section on problems with eating in Chapter 3. In a sample of 230 children and adults seen at our center, one-third had had, during childhood, very limited diets—for example, eating only dried spaghetti—and there was a real worry about their health. Surprisingly, few if any of these children showed signs of malnutrition. Another third had marked food fads but did eat enough for adequate nutrition. Nearly one third had excessive intake of fluids during childhood. Retention of bowel contents for a week or more was reported during childhood for about 12 percent and minor problems of this kind for another 12 percent. We have only recently started to collect data about loose and frequent bowel movements, so detailed information is not available. The difficulty is to know how to interpret these observations. I agree with the view that many food fads and retention of bowel movements are manifestations of repetitive routines. Some feeding problems, especially those involving refusal of food needing chewing, arise from difficulties in coordinating the movements of chewing and swallowing. However, there are workers who believe all these behaviors indicate pathology in the gastrointestinal tract, and they incorporate this view into their theories of the causes of autistic disorders, as described below.

Infections and MMR Vaccination

Viral infections of the mother, such as rubella, in the early stages of pregnancy, or viral infections in the young child complicated by encephalitis, which can happen with, for example, mumps and measles, are occasional causes of autistic disorders. This is of particular interest because, at the time of this writing, there is great concern that the triple vaccine against measles, mumps and rubella (MMR) may be the cause of autistic disorders in some children. One team of research workers has reported finding abnormalities of the lymphoid tissue, containing the measles virus, in the lining of the intestines in children whose parents believe that autism began after MMR vaccination. They attribute the feeding and bowel problems to this. Their findings have not, so far, been confirmed by other investigators.

The apparent rise in prevalence reported in recent years has been cited in support of the theory that MMR can cause autistic disorders. The prevalence rates found over the years and possible reasons for the reported rise are discussed in Chapter 4. The weight of the evidence suggests that the rise is due to wider diagnostic criteria and improved recognition rather than a real change. In any case, careful studies of trends in numbers have shown no relationship in time with the introduction of MMR vaccination.

The problem for parents of children with autism is that MMR vaccination is usually given around the time when they begin to notice unusual behavior in their child. The early signs of problems in the first year of life are often not noticed by parents, who then think that the autism began later, perhaps after the MMR vaccination. Because of the recent publicity, parents of young children now need good evidence to convince them that the benefits of vaccination far outweigh the small risks inherent in any medical procedure. Some parents want their children to receive the three vaccinations singly, with an interval between, but this increases the likelihood of a child being infected while waiting for the next single vaccination. The irony is that infections with measles, mumps and rubella can all have serious consequences, including autistic disorders.

Allergy

Some parents and professionals believe that autistic disorders are autoimmune conditions or are caused by allergy to, for example, fungal infections, virus infections, vaccinations or various foods. They consider that the feeding and bowel problems are part of the allergic picture. Treatments based on such theories have been followed by some families. The results reported have varied from positive to negative but there has been no properly controlled evaluation.

Biochemical Abnormalities and Diet

The levels in bodily fluids of various neurotransmitters and hormones have been investigated in cases of autistic disorders but results tend to be inconsistent. The most definite finding is of raised levels of the neurotransmitter serotonin as measured in the blood in about one-quarter of individuals with autism, although low serotonin levels can also be found in a few autistic individuals. Raised serotonin also occurs in a disparate collection of other conditions so its relevance in autism is still not clear. The drug fenfluramine was given to children with autism because it lowers serotonin levels but the results were disappointing.

There has been much interest in the family of peptides that are neuroregulators known as opioids, meaning morphine-like. One current theory contends that autism results from excessive levels of opioids in the brain, leading to autistic features including reduced pain sensitivity, lessening of social behavior, increased stereotypies and lowering of appetite and bowel movements. It is suggested that abnormalities of the gastrointestinal tract in autistic people could increase permeability of the intestinal wall and allow the large peptide molecules to pass into the blood stream and from there to the brain. Peptides from milk, wheat and some other cereals have opioid-like activity. From this it is argued that autism can be treated with a casein- and gluten-free diet. There are anecdotal reports of good results from diets of this kind. There are also reports of no change and others where the parents found it so hard to ensure that the child kept to the diet and the child found the food so unpleasant that the trial was abandoned. I know of no properly controlled trials and without these it is impossible to evaluate the results.

Some people recommend the administration of high doses of vitamins, such as the B complex, and of various minerals. Again, there are both positive and negative reports of the results and the value of this approach is controversial.

Secretin

Secretin is a hormone that, among other functions, stimulates the pancreas to produce substances that aid the process of digestion. It is used in tests of pancreatic function. In the mid-1990s there was a report from a parent that her son who had autism showed remarkable improvement after being given secretin. It was suggested that the pancreatic enzymes stimulated by secretin would help break down peptides that could cause autistic behavior, thus leading to improvement. There was no direct evidence for this hypothesis. The other effects of secretin, including actions on the brain, were also considered as possible explanations. The most important question to be answered was whether this hormone was really effective in improving autistic behavior. Anecdotal reports were both positive and negative. The hormone had to be given by intravenous infusion under medical supervision and had to be carefully monitored, so all kinds of possible adverse effects needed to be considered. In any event, the few controlled trials conducted so far have failed to show more improvement from the secretin than from the placebo.

The Pathology in the Brain

How and where do the original causes, including genetic factors, affect the brain? Do all types of causes home in on the same brain structures and functions or are there different pathological pictures that can all give rise to autistic behavior? Do different subgroups of autistic symptoms correspond to different types of brain dysfunctions?

Evidence is being sought from post-mortem studies and brain imaging techniques in life. Such studies have suggested various brain areas that may be involved, including the brain stem, the temporal lobe, the limbic system, the cerebellum and the frontal lobe. Currently there is much interest in the amygdala. There is evidence that a proportion of children with autistic disorders have unusually large head circumferences and post-mortem studies have found some with large brains.

A 1966 study of five young adults with Asperger syndrome used PET (positron emission tomography) scans to examine an area in the left medial prefrontal cortex of their brains. Other studies had shown this area of the brain to be active in volunteers without

Asperger syndrome or other signs of atypical development when they performed tasks requiring them to consider what might be going on in another person's mind (the "Theory of Mind" tests— see below). In those with Asperger syndrome, no activity was observed in this part of the brain during the task, though other areas were active. The exact mechanisms and pathways leading to this finding have still to be elucidated.

Research is also continuing on the neurochemicals involved in transmission of messages in the brain, and on physiological measures of brain activity. Also of interest to researchers are hormones, such as oxytocin, that affect early brain development.

The difficulty faced by investigators of brain pathology in autistic disorders essentially comes down to the complexity of brain development and brain function. The interaction between different parts of the brain and the way the functions of each part are influenced by others is still far from being understood and mapped. So far there have been no consistent findings concerning brain structure and function in autistic disorders. The published studies fail to corroborate previous findings or even contradict each other. The reason may be that there are many different paths that can lead to an autistic disorder and many different patterns of neuropathology. The subgroups of autistic disorders may not be identifiable from the overt clinical picture, so different studies may actually be examining different subgroups—of questionable relevance to some other subgroups or to the overall spectrum of symptoms and causes—even when they try to make them compatible on clinical criteria. Nevertheless, advances in brain imaging techniques are likely to occur, and these hold out the best hope of solving the mystery of autism.

Psychological Dysfunctions

All kinds of studies of different aspects of psychological dysfunctions have been carried out in the attempt to identify the nature of the impairment, or impairments, that underlie the characteristic autistic behavior, especially the triad of impairments. These include investigations of language, memory, attention and visuo-spatial skills. The most recent development in this area has come from the studies on the growth in normal children's understanding of other people's thoughts and feelings. This developmental skill is referred to as the "theory of mind." Uta Frith and Simon Baron-Cohen and their colleagues investigated this in children with autism of the kind described by Kanner and found marked impairments. This fits well with the typical social indifference of young children with autism and with the social naivete of the older, more able individuals. In normal development, theory of mind does not emerge until three to four years of age. Its impairment in children with autistic disorders presumably has its roots in their lack of interest in social interaction, which is detectable very early in life.

With further investigation, complications became evident—a familiar experience in research. The developmental level of theory of mind, even in autism, is related to language comprehension. Some children can pass the simpler tests, though are defeated by more complex theory of mind tasks. When young adults with the pattern described by Asperger or with high-functioning autism are tested, some are able to pass all the tests although they show a marked lack of understanding of other people in real-life situations. The PET scan study mentioned above suggests that people with Asperger's syndrome or high-functioning autism use a different part of the brain than most people to try to solve theory of mind tests. This works in artificial "laboratory" tests but not in real-life situations. As Uta Frith has pointed out, the tests of theory of mind that have been devised to date are designed for research and should not be used for diagnosis of autistic conditions. Passing these tests does not rule out the diagnosis. More sophisticated tests need to be developed to reveal the precise nature of the social impairment.

Some researchers consider that the primary roots of autism lie in absence or impairment of built-in social instinct, present from birth. There is no doubt that problems of social interaction are seen very early in most children with autistic disorders. It seems likely that people with autistic disorders have great difficulty in seeing, or rather feeling, meaning in their experiences. Instead of developing the usual pattern of priorities that are common to humanity (though modified by culture), only a few things have emotional significance for people with autistic disorders and these tend to be idiosyncratic to the person concerned and usually of little use in adapting to life. The research into how the brain assigns significance to objects and events may prove to be of great relevance to autistic disorders.

Four problems have to be considered in relation to all research in this field. First, because autistic disorders can be associated with various conditions affecting the brain, the abnormalities that are specific to autism have to be distinguished from others that may be present. Second, the problems related to autism have to be separated from those due to any associated learning difficulties. This is difficult because learning difficulties can occur as a consequence of autistic disorders as well as from other conditions that may be present and that may or may not be linked with the autism. Third, the features, such as odd responses to sensory stimuli and motor problems, that are very common in autistic disorders but are not considered essential for diagnosis, also have to be accounted for in any comprehensive theory of causation. Fourth, the difficulties of definition of autistic disorders make it hard to compare studies. Interview and observation schedules have been designed to obtain detailed clinical information to aid in ensuring comparability between samples of subjects used for research. These are helpful but, as discussed above, do not entirely solve the problems. Much of the research to date has concentrated on children who have autism of the Kanner type. More recently, those with the behavior described by Asperger have been investigated. It would be interesting and helpful to extend research to cover all those with the triad of impairments and to include adults of all ages as well as children. Another approach to research in the field would be to compare the pathology in autistic disorders with that in conditions, such as Fragile X, in which some but not all aspects of the autistic picture are found.

PART II

Living with Autistic Disorders

CHAPTER 7

Problems Faced by Parents

Parents have to cope with a series of problems, some of which are practical and some of which are emotional. Many of these are common to parents of children with any kind of disability, while others are special to the families of children with autistic disorders.

The parents of any child with a long-term disability have to undergo a change of attitude when they first learn the truth and this is a painful process. Like all parents, they start off with the expectation that they have a perfect baby who will grow up to be a fully independent adult. They have to adjust to the fact that all their hopes and plans for their child's future, and their own future as well, will have to be changed.

They may have feelings of guilt, which are a waste of mental energy that can be turned to better use. Professional workers can help parents to develop a constructive attitude. The workers who fail to diagnose an autistic disorder and attribute the strange behavior to parental mishandling, or recognize autism but consider that it is caused by the parents, do great harm to the families and the children. Such ideas are gradually becoming less common but still exist.

Autistic disorders in a child cause special emotional problems for parents. The disability is not detectable at birth and is rarely diagnosed before 18 months. Parents go through emotional swings, at times knowing that something is wrong and at other times persuading themselves that all is well.

They reassure themselves because the child's physical development gives no cause for alarm and, every now and again, the child

does something so skillfully that it seems they must be highly intelligent. On the other hand, social aloofness, when it is present, is
painful and baffling for the parents. It is a common experience for
parents to feel that there must be one simple key, which, if found
could solve all the problems. Eventually the anxiety they have been
feeling is seen to be justified and a professional opinion is sought.
By this time the parents have swung so often between hope and
despair that they may find the truth hard to accept.

Before the diagnosis is made parents often feel they are the only
people in the world to have a child with such strange behavior and
the knowledge that there are many others comes as a great relief.
Meeting other parents through local autism groups is a source of
emotional and practical support. The experience of emotional isolation in the child's early years is becoming less common as knowledge of autistic disorders increases, but it still occurs. This is one
of the major reasons for the importance of early and accurate diagnosis. Research into ways of identifying the basic impairments
early in life is ongoing and progress is being made.

In the early years of a child with an autistic disorder, the parents' attachment makes them persevere, even if the child shows
little or no response. Despite all the difficulties, the very weakness
and dependence of a child with a disability tends to make the natural attachment of parent to child even stronger. This attachment
has positive results in that the child is loved and cared for. When
progress does occur, each small step forward is all the more rewarding because it was so long in coming. The negative side is the
tendency to give less attention to the other members of the family
who are more independent but still need their parents' love and
support.

Helping a child with an autistic disorder to develop skills and
enjoy activities is hard work and time consuming. Combining this
with bringing up other children as well sounds like an impossible
feat. The only solution is to organize a routine so that each member of the family has their fair share of the parents' attention. A short
session with a parent regularly each day is better than longer ses-

sions occurring sporadically. Parents should not forget *themselves* in their timetable. They need some rest and relaxation away from the family in order to preserve their sense of proportion. If their horizons are limited exclusively to the daily life of the child who is disabled, no one benefits, least of all the child concerned.

Children with autistic disorders can cause parents extra expense if they destroy clothing, furniture, windows, wallpaper and so forth. If they are not toilet trained, diapers have to be provided and sheets and other bedding continually washed. Depending upon the parents' income, the nature and severity of a child's disability, and other factors, parents may qualify for some type of financial assistance from the government such as Supplemental Security Income (SSI).

The social life of the family tends to be restricted by a child with a disability, especially an autistic disorder. If the children are behaviorally disturbed, it may be difficult to find babysitters and the parents may never be able to go out together. Some parent support groups may have a scheme for babysitting. If not, then the idea can be suggested and explored by interested members. Such schemes are always the result of individual initiatives.

Taking the child out in public can lead to problems. Most of them show no evidence of disability in their appearance. If they behave oddly, some strangers are critical and assume the child is "spoiled." A sensitive parent may avoid taking out the child, even on expeditions they might enjoy. For the sake of the child and the whole family, parents have to develop thick skins and take the child out as much as possible, ignoring the stares of the ill-educated. Teaching appropriate behavior in public, beginning as early as possible, does help to reduce the major problems (see Chapter 11). Public awareness of and sympathy for people with autistic disorders has greatly increased since the first edition of this book was written, helped by publicity in the media and the film *Rain Man*.

Most parents are concerned about having another child, especially if the one with an autistic disorder is their first. There is now strong evidence that there is a raised risk of parents having more than one child with an autistic disorder unless the cause in the first child is known and is clearly not genetic. Parents have to consider the facts as they relate to themselves and their families and make their own decisions.

The problems of other children in the family who themselves are developing normally are discussed in Chapter 8. These add to the parents' concerns. If siblings ask questions about autistic disorders, including the risk to themselves of having a child who is also affected, the best strategy is for parents to answer the questions with honesty when asked. Some families find Sandra Harris' book, *Siblings of Children with Autism: A Guide for Families,* to be helpful in these instances.

Relatives often provide help and support. Grandparents, for example, can be a major source of emotional and practical help, including babysitting. Loving grandparents may develop a special relationship with the autistic child, somehow finding a way around the social and communication impairments.

Unhappily, the attitudes of some relatives may be less constructive. They may feel that a child with a disability reflects badly on the whole family, thus disregarding the fact that all families have relatives with disabilities somewhere in their histories. They may try to lay the blame on one or other parent or their ancestry. They may reject the child and try to avoid seeing them or involving them in family affairs, visits or outings. Equally distressing is the relative who insists that there is nothing wrong with the child and that all the problems are due to the parents' methods of child-rearing and dealing with difficult behavior. The best way to cope with this attitude is to keep cool, calm and dignified, provide information but refuse to be drawn into arguments. If there is no other way of changing attitudes, visit as little as possible with those who are unsympathetic.

It cannot be emphasized too strongly that autistic children vary widely in the severity of their disabilities and in the amount of progress they can make—ranging from very little all the way to the achievement of independence in adult life. The parents of the children with the most severe disabilities have to cope with the sadness of seeing little improvement in their own child, while knowing others with autistic disorders have made great strides. When the diagnosis is first made, all parents hope that their own child will be one of those with a good prognosis, but follow-up studies have shown that a substantial number of children are not in this category. This is just one more hard fact among many with which parents have to come to terms. It is pointless for them to waste time in blaming themselves for their child's problems. The constructive approach is to aim to find a way of life for their disabled child in which he will be as happy and content as possible, whatever his level of function. Parents whose children make good progress should avoid taking a superior attitude to others whose children do less well. When the children grow up, the parents of those who are more able often have to watch without being able to help while their sons or daughters try to become independent and suffer in the process. The parents of those with more severe disabilities who will be dependent on others all their lives are at least saved this source of distress.

Parents with children who will never become independent as adults worry about what will happen to their child when they themselves can no longer care for them. The practical steps parents can take are to ensure that the child is known to the local social services, to investigate different types of residential accommodations well before this becomes essential, and to obtain legal advice concerning wills and trusts if this is appropriate to the family's financial situation.

Unity within the family is a major factor in coping successfully with the strain of raising a child with an autistic disorder. It is important to avoid the temptation to blame the other partner for the child's behavior. It does no good, and a lot of harm, to criticize each other for mishandling the child. Discussions concerning genetic traits in the family are interesting if pursued in the spirit of intellectual inquiry but not if they are used as the focus of blame.

A series of sleepless nights and terrible days can try the patience of a saint, but the effort to remain calm and reasonable is well worthwhile. Keeping one's temper and refusing to nag or become irritable all become easier if worked at consistently. Good family relations have a beneficial effect on the child's behavior, in part because any child is happier and easier to manage within a united family. Also, the proper handling of difficult behavior demands a consistent approach from both parents who must back each other's decisions in front of the child and reserve questions and discussions on methods for when they are alone together.

Some parents are drawn closer together by the experience of having a child with a disability, while others are torn apart by the stress. Support from relatives on both sides of the family, help from professional workers and appropriate placements in preschools, schools and adult services all contribute to lessening the burdens on families. A sense of humor is also a great help. Many of the things that the children do and say are extremely funny, even if trying at the time they happen, and it does one good to laugh at them in retrospect.

Occasionally one is faced with the dilemma of knowing another family with a child who probably has an autistic disorder but whose parents are unaware or unwilling to face the possibility. If the child's parents do not know about autism, tactful inquiries and comments may prove to be the catalyst needed for the family to begin to find help. If on the other hand the parents do not want to know, there is nothing that can be done except to wait until they begin to acknowledge there is a problem and to be ready with help at the right moment.

CHAPTER 8

Sisters and Brothers

Studies on the effects on children of living with a sibling with various kinds of disabilities, including autistic disorders, have offered conflicting results. It seems that some children are adversely affected whereas others cope well. The effects are related to a series of definable and indefinable factors, including the severity of the disability, whether or not the child has disturbed behavior, the personalities of the brothers and sisters and the attitudes of the parents.

Those children with siblings with autistic disorders do face a number of special problems. Perhaps the hardest thing for them is that their parents have to give so much time and attention to the special child that there is little to spare for the rest of the family. This is particularly likely to affect a sister or brother who is close in age to the child with the disability. Parents need to be aware of this danger and do their best to set aside time for their other children and to show them that they are equally loved and valued. If it is possible to arrange for some domestic help, this may enable the parents to organize their time more easily.

A destructive autistic child may break toys and other things. Brothers and sisters need to have a special safe place to lock away their precious possessions and, if possible, a room of their own. If possible, parents should replace damaged possessions and try to teach children with autistic disorders not to touch any objects except their own. If sisters and brothers are reassured that their rights are being respected, they are likely to accept the occasional loss of a possession with better grace.

School-age siblings may feel uncomfortable bringing their friends home to play. If at all possible, parents should encourage friends to visit. It is best to explain about autism frankly and simply and to answer the questions of the brothers and sisters and their friends in as calm and relaxed a manner as possible. The child with the autistic disorder may be able to play with the others but if they habitually disrupt activities parents should try to arrange for their other children and friends to have some time to themselves.

Many children enjoy playing with and teaching their siblings with autistic disorders and can involve them in a variety of activities. Brothers and sisters are often more successful in this than their parents. Children with a sibling who is disabled in any way often develop a level of maturity beyond their years and many go into the caring professions in adult life.

Parents of children with autistic disorders have to beware of placing too much responsibility on the shoulders of their other children and to make sure that they have plenty of time for their own pursuits. Parents are naturally concerned about the future of their disabled child and some may hope that a sister or brother will eventually take on the responsibility of care. This is a hard burden to place on young shoulders and could, if taken seriously by the sibling, disadvantage them throughout their life. It is best to let brothers and sisters make their own decisions as to how much involvement they can sustain rather than subjecting them to emotional pressure—overt or covert.

There are some brothers or sisters who find it hard to interact with a child with an autistic disorder. Their feelings should be respected and they should not be pressured to be involved or made to feel guilty. This can be hard advice for a parent who is desperate for help—but a reluctant, resentful helper is worse than no helper at all.

Before they understand the nature of autism, the siblings may worry about the possibility of themselves developing autistic behavior. They may have all kinds of alarming fears and fantasies and parents need to be sensitive to these feelings. They can help by their calm acceptance of all their children, their willingness to discuss and explain the situation and offer their love and reassurance.

Adolescents are often concerned about the possibility of their own future children having autistic disorders. As discussed in Chapter 6, there is an increased risk of another child with an autistic disorder, or with more subtle autistic traits, being born to parents who already have one child with typical autism. The precise risk of siblings having a child with the same type of disability has not been calculated but it seems likely that it is higher than that for the general population. The exact risk varies depending on the cause. For example, if it is known that the cause of autism was rubella during the mother's pregnancy, genetic factors are much less likely to be a factor. Put the matter into perspective; explain that there are many different conditions in addition to autistic disorders that can produce congenital disabilities and few families have no such problems in their past histories.

The journal of the British National Autistic Society, *Communication*, publishes occasional articles by sisters and brothers of children or adults with autistic disorders. Some find it helpful to meet or correspond with others in the same situation and can make contacts through the society.

CHAPTER 9

Making Sense of Time and Space

Autistic disorders affect all activities of daily living and they are usually lifelong, even in those who markedly improve. There is no known cure for these disabilities, but this does not mean that nothing can be done. Those affected with autism can be helped to compensate for their difficulties by utilizing special methods of education, both at home and at school. In many ways the problems are similar to those faced by parents and teachers of children with hearing or visual impairments that cannot be cured. The children can be helped through education to develop their full potential, however large or small this may be. Adults can be given the opportunities to make the best use of the skills they do possess. Some of the children have too many additional disabilities to make much progress but, even in these cases, it is worth trying to encourage more appropriate behavior and to teach simple self-care. For those who are more able, much can be achieved.

In many ways, the learning difficulties and inappropriate behavior found in autistic spectrum disorders are similar to those found in other developmental disabilities and many of the general principles underlying methods of teaching and caring can be applied. However, the basic autistic inability to make sense of past and present experiences leads to special difficulties in comprehending time and space. These specific difficulties must be understood and taken into account if programs and caring are to be successful. In the rest of this book many more examples of problems of time and space, and suggestions for ways of helping, will be provided under different headings. However, this aspect of the autistic disorders is so important for understanding how the children and adults see the world it needs an entire chapter.

The problems with time are not related to telling time by the clock, which some people with autistic disorders are able to do well. The difficulties lie in comprehending the passage of time and linking it with ongoing activities. This often shows itself as an inability to wait. Impatience is common in all young children, but in people with autistic disorders it can continue for years, even into adult life. Some begin to scream if made to wait more than a second for their food, for a walk, for a ride in the car or for anything else they want.

Another aspect of poor understanding of time is seen when trying to persuade a child to wash, dress and generally prepare for school or some other event within the time available. Even the most able individuals may find it impossible to cope with time limits, which can be a major barrier to becoming independent.

One of the most obvious examples of confusion with time is the way in which those with enough speech continually ask for re-assurance about future events and when they will happen. They want to have the timetable spelled out in precise detail, not once but an infinite number of times. Parents and teachers are tempted to ascribe this to a desire for attention or to be annoying but the underlying anxiety associated with the questions shows that there is a real difficulty in understanding that the future will eventually become the present.

Another aspect of this problem is the lack of awareness that an event, once started, will come to an end. Some children have been extremely distressed when taken on a new expedition because they did not know if they would ever return home again and did not have the words to ask. The fear generated by being lost in time also explains why there is often such a strong adverse reaction to any unpredictable change in the expected timetable. Some more-able children who can tell time by the clock become obsessed with time and demand that everything happens at the precise pre-ordained moment. Woe betide the parent of such a child who promises to do something in "just five minutes" and then takes six minutes and 14 seconds.

The trouble with time is that it cannot be seen or felt but has to be inferred from the sequence of events. There is some similarity with speech, which has no visible, tangible form and has gone as soon as the words have been uttered. It seems that people with autistic disorders have severe problems with coping with sequential events that have no independent, concrete existence. Concepts of time have always puzzled and fascinated philosophers but most people are born with the ability to understand it in everyday terms. People with autistic disorders seem to lack this understanding to a degree that is markedly discrepant with their level of intelligence.

The best way to help an autistic person is to represent the passage of time in practical terms—the abstract has to be made concrete. Visual timetables are invaluable. They can be composed of drawings, photographs, words if the child can read, or a combination of these. The days can be divided into segments marked by meal and snack times. The sequence of time can be shown by the progression of days from left to right, in countries where this is the convention for writing. Each child should have their own timetable. The day can begin with the child going through the pictured events of that day with the help of a parent or teacher. Some children like to mark the previous day to show that it has gone. When talking through the timetable, the end of each event should be explained as well as its beginning—"After lunch we shall go to the park and play on the swings. Then we shall come back home again." When setting out on any expedition, it should be made clear that it will end in a return home or other base.

Such timetables are useful for introducing planned changes into the program. Unplanned changes should be avoided if at all possible. If they do happen on short notice, as much explanation and reassurance as possible should be given. Some children like to have any unexpected changes inserted into their personal timetable as a record of the past that they can talk about afterwards. The timetables should be kept so that they can be used to talk about the past as well as the future. This can be a source of much pleasure for some children. Parents often say how sad it is that their children do not seem to recall happy events, or to look forward to enjoyable occasions, especially Christmas or other special festivals, because this means they lack two of the major sources of pleasure in life. Making and keeping records of past and future events helps to develop appreciation of past pleasures and those to come. Photographs, slides and videos can all be used for this purpose.

The passing of shorter periods of time can also be marked by cues. A child can be helped to stay on task or to wait quietly for something to happen if the end of the time allotted or the waiting period is marked in some way. Unless the child can tell time by the clock it is not usually possible for them to comprehend that time is moving by looking at either a digital or an analogue clock. It is easier for them if the end of a time period is marked with an alarm or kitchen timer. Alternatively, time can be made visible by using a device like the computer method of showing the progress of a program by gradually coloring in a long rectangle.

More-able children also need assistance in organizing themselves. The problems are particularly acute in mainstream school. Personal timetables, written lists (for example, the things they have to take to school each day), written instructions and maps to show them when and where to go if they have lessons in more than one classroom can ease their way through school. Someone to whom they can always turn for help and who understands the reasons for their confusion is essential. The same kind of help is needed for autistic adults.

People with autistic disorders also have problems understanding boundaries and relationships between objects in space. Among the very young and those who are severely disabled, there may be confusion about the parts of their own bodies. For example, a five-year-old girl with autism still regarded her own hand emerging from a sleeve as if she had never seen it before. The children may find it hard to relate images of the same object seen from different points of view, which may explain why they often closely examine objects from different angles. They may be unaware of the boundaries between objects that to others seem so obvious. For example, they may not know where their own house ends and the next one begins. They are usually quite unaware of the subtle boundaries that are not physically marked, such as other people's personal space, or the areas on the crowded beach occupied by other families. It is not surprising that they are baffled by the complex relationships between people.

To help reduce the confusion, boundaries in space and time and relationships between people, objects and events have to be explained in as simple a way as possible using every available way of expressing concepts in visual terms. An album of photographs of familiar places can be used as a teaching aid. Looking through the pictures every day, naming things in them and retelling stories of events involving the child is an activity that many of the children enjoy. It is a useful substitute for a bedtime story for those who are not interested in fiction.

People with autistic disorders lack an internal structure for their lives. They need to have an external framework constructed for them by those who care for them and teach them. Even those who are most able need this type of support. The most successful find it for themselves in the work and living arrangements they choose, but even they are vulnerable if the structure is completely removed by the hazards of life.

Whatever you do in this life, there is always a down side. In this case the disadvantage is that when a child with an autistic disorder appreciates and is helped by a timetable, it can become a repetitive routine that must not be changed under any circumstances. Using the technique to introduce changes deliberately helps to overcome this. Despite possible problems, the positive gains of using timetables outweigh the negative aspects.

CHAPTER 10

The Triad of Impairments

The cluster of impairments of social interaction, communication and imagination and the consequent repetitive pattern of behavior is the common thread connecting all autistic disorders, whatever other conditions may be present. Teachers with training and experience in the field are developing methods of helping children to compensate for their disabilities and a range of books and papers is available. The aim is to give some simple ideas that parents can use in everyday situations.

Social Interaction

This is the aspect of autistic conditions that causes parents the most heartache and feelings of inadequacy and guilt that are totally undeserved.

DEVELOPING SOCIAL CONTACT

The young child with typical autism of the kind described by Kanner appears aloof and indifferent to others and happy in his or her own world unless someone interferes. One of the barriers to making contact with such a child can be his or her dislike of being touched. This can make washing and dressing a nightmare and cause the child to resist being held by the hand when out walking. Paradoxically, the children usually enjoy rough-and-tumble play and this can be used to give them the feeling that contact with other people can be enjoyable. The play sessions can begin with more active play and then gradually become quieter and gentler. This type of contact can be associated with other experiences that are enjoyed, such as a mid-morning drink or cookie. If the child likes music, as so many of them do, they may be happy to sit on a parent's lap and be rocked while listening to a favorite tune. They may be more receptive to this after some physical activity or after a bath. It may be necessary to start with only a few seconds of contact and then gradually to increase the time.

Some aspects of appropriate social behavior can be taught, even though they are used in a mechanical way. Eye contact does tend to improve with increasing age but it can be encouraged. Providing this does not cause distress, the child's head can be gently held to attract their visual attention when talking to them. Some will make eye contact if the adult makes funny faces, or sings a favorite song. One game that a little girl enjoyed was touching noses with her mother who then twisted her head to create a funny visual effect. The child happily made eye contact to ask for this game and then used it for other requests.

Positive signs of affection within the family can also be taught. Instead of allowing the child to accept a hug and a kiss passively, their own arms can be guided to return the hug. It is best for the child to learn this as a response to affection from others rather than encouraging them to initiate the contact, in case they assume that this is the way to greet everyone.

A child can be taught to shake hands if their hand is guided correctly whenever a visitor offers a hand first. Again, it is better to teach this as a response to a proffered hand rather than encouraging the child to make the first move because they will not understand when it is correct to do this and when it is not. With the children who can speak, teaching polite behavior, such as saying "please" and "thank you," is worthwhile. They have no idea why people do this but it helps to make them more socially acceptable.

Although they lack the built-in social instinct, the children do, in the course of time, become attached in their own way to the people who care for them. This is partly due to the fact that their parents or other caregivers become familiar to them and partly because they provide the things the child wants. This is "cupboard love" to start with but it does grow into something deeper over the years. It is never the same as instinctive feelings but it is no less genuine. The attachment grows most easily if parents are calm and consistent in their approach, provide a clear framework of rules that apply to all family members and give the child some pleasant experiences to make up for the fact that ordinary life tends to be a constant source of anxiety and confusion for them.

Sisters and brothers, especially if they are of an age at which they are willing and eager to play, also become important to a child with an autistic disorder. Often the sibling leads the child with an autistic disorder into all kinds of activities in which they would not otherwise engage. The fact that the child is mostly or always a passive partner does not matter. The experience of play is of benefit.

Even if they relate well to siblings, it is easier for autistic children to relate to adults than to children outside the family, especially those of the same age. This is probably because adults are able to adapt themselves to the child whereas other children, unless they also have siblings who are autistic, do not have the necessary insight and do not modify their behavior. Most children with autistic disorders with moderate or severe handicaps will always need adult supervision and guidance whenever they are with a group of same-age children. They must be protected from bullying and teasing. Children with autistic disorders cannot defend themselves and do not learn to do so through experience. They have neither the verbal wit nor the physical skills to hold their own among their peers. The situation must never be allowed to degenerate so that the autistic child reacts with random aggression, or else withdraws and wanders away on his own.

So far I have concentrated upon ways of encouraging social mixing. The other side of the picture can be seen in some children who make good progress. They may become over-friendly and sociable in an immature way and fail to discriminate between people they know and complete strangers. One ten-year-old girl would rush up to strangers with a joyful greeting, often to their amazement. Her parents had to restrain her and explain many times over that she must not talk to people in the street unless her parents make the first move. She was most upset at first, but the phase passed after a few months. There is no easy answer since parents do not want to discourage a spontaneous friendliness that they have spent so long in encouraging. However, I have not met any children who have become withdrawn again because their over-friendliness has had to be curbed.

Expeditions, Vacations and Social Occasions

Trips out with parents, brothers and sisters are a part of family so-cial life. Young children with autistic disorders often find crowds and bustle confusing and frightening. At this stage, family expedi-tions should be carefully planned. They should be kept fairly short and not too far from home so that it is easy to remove the child if the situation proves too distressing. Different kinds of outings can be tried. If one is not a success then it is best to leave it for a while and try again later. A visit to the zoo, with lively, noisy, smelly an-imals, may terrify a young child but be enjoyed when the child is older. When the child is able to understand, they can be prepared in advance by explaining in words and pictures where they are going, what will happen there, how long it will last and, very impor-tantly, that they will in the end return home. Details such as when and where they will eat and whether there are toilets, and if not, how they will cope, have to be included in the story.

Most young children with autistic disorders do not under-stand the point of birthday parties and do not participate if parents invite other children. There is no point in trying to make them take part in such events. Older and more-able children may like to go to parties although they may not join in. One boy who liked sitting and watching the other children at parties was sad when his sisters were invited without him. The hosts had not realized that in his own quiet way he was enjoying himself. Parents, who so often have to stand between the world and their child, need to overcome any diffidence they feel and explain to friends and relations about their child's condition so that the child has as much social life as possi-ble. When the family entertains, the child with an autistic disorder may enjoy having a special role, such as passing dishes of nuts or candy, or clearing the table after the meal. This has to be practiced in advance and the guests need to be primed to express praise and appreciation if this pleases the child.

Although some children with autistic disorders are afraid of trains or buses, many love traveling in any form of transport and may be calmer and happier when on the move than in any other situation. However, apart from the actual journey, vacations away from home may be difficult. A young child may be bewildered by new surroundings and may never settle down during the period away from home. Many families do not take a vacation, or else try to arrange temporary residential care for the child while the rest of the family goes away. The problems often lessen as the child grows older. A short break should be tried first. A self-catering vacation away from other people has obvious advantages.

As always, advance preparation using pictures to explain exactly what will happen makes all the difference to the children who can understand. Some of the child's favorite possessions should be taken and the activities planned so that the child is kept amused and happy as much as possible. The aim is to associate going away on vacation with happy occasions so that eventually trips become easier to organize. The effort is worthwhile because new experiences that the child enjoys help to build confidence in place of fear. One child found it difficult to tolerate a long journey the first time this was tried. She had no idea how long the journey would take and what would happen at the end, despite the parents' attempts to explain. She was able to recognize and match written words so that on the next long journey she was given a list of all the towns on the route. The signs with the names on them were pointed out and she crossed them off her list as they were passed. This proved an enjoyable occupation and showed her, in visual terms, the length of the journey.

Communication

In the first edition of this book, I included a description of a method intended to teach children with autistic disorders to speak that was used by psychologists who advocated the "operant conditioning" approach. Briefly, the technique was gradually to "shape" the sounds made by the child by rewarding nearer and nearer approximations to words. Even then, there was considerable doubt as to the effectiveness of this system. Now it is clear that the language impairments in autistic disorders are primarily due to the lack of the normally innate drive to communicate with others. There may or may not be developmental language disorders in addition to this fundamental impairment but the communication problems cannot be overcome simply by teaching the children to speak, even if that were possible.

Within the autistic spectrum, including those who are most able, the majority of children do develop speech sooner or later and most do so without specialist help. The problem is that this speech is based on a vocabulary that is learned by rote, although those who make the most progress do become fluent with a large store of words. The best way for parents to try to encourage the communicative use of speech is to give the child as wide a range as possible of social and other experiences. Preparing in advance with words and pictures and retelling events afterwards with more words and pictures provide the opportunity for the child to make connections between events and to learn that words have meanings in the real world. If a video camera is available, videotapes of special occasions are useful for gaining the attention of some children. Even if videos can be made, still photographs have their advantages as well because they capture one single moment in time. The ordinary events of everyday life as well as special trips and treats provide plenty of material for these sessions. This type of interaction with parents and siblings helps the children to develop some awareness that talking to others can be interesting and rewarding.

The abnormalities of speech that are characteristic of autistic disorders were described in Chapter 3. It is not helpful to correct these odd ways of speaking. It is more important to encourage the child to communicate in whatever way they can. Where appropriate, rephrasing the child's utterances when replying without criticizing is more useful.

In contrast to the children who speak very little, there are some who talk repetitively and far too much. Their speech is not used for two-way communication. The same ideas for enlarging experiences and using them to develop understanding are just as relevant for these children.

For children with no or very limited speech, the signs the child does use, such as indicating by touching or pointing, should be encouraged. If a child has no other means of expressing their needs, it is preferable for them to lead someone by the arm to show what is wanted than to scream. At this stage the parent can teach the child by repetition to respond to the words "show me" while putting out a hand to be taken. Every opportunity should be taken to reward more appropriate methods of communicating, but any method is better than nothing. Teaching a manual sign language, such as the Makaton system, can be tried although, almost always, the same limitations and abnormalities are found in signed as in spoken speech. Occasionally a child learns to use signs much better than speech. Presumably this occurs when the child has an additional developmental disorder affecting expressive speech but has sufficient inner language to allow them to express more in signs. For this reason it is always worth trying to teach a sign language, but the child should not be pressured to use it if there is little or no progress.

Imagination

Pretend play is the earliest indicator of the development of imagination. Like speech, it is either conspicuous by its absence, or repetitive if present. Some children will learn a sequence of actions, such as preparing, pouring out and offering a pretend cup of tea, but true creativity in play, especially that shared with other children, cannot be taught. Sometimes sisters or brothers involve the children in pretend games, assigning them a role they can carry out as directed.

The children who have repetitive "pretend" play, including acting out scenes from videos or other sources, do have a way of occupying themselves, which can be a relief for parents. If the child becomes so involved in one activity that it takes over from all other activities, then limiting the time spent on such play is necessary. This does involve parents in the task of finding other activities to replace the repetitive play.

The value of true imagination and creativity is in associating past and present experiences and making plans for the future— ranging from the mundane what to do tomorrow to the grand plans for the whole of life. The impairment of this aspect of development in people with autistic disorders is a constantly repeated theme throughout this book because it has such wide and deep implications for their lives. Ways of helping the children to conceptualize past, present and future by representing them in visual terms have been described in Chapter 9.

Resistance to Change and Repetitive Activities

This type of behavior ranks high on the list of problems that cause parents the most worry and despair. If not handled properly, a child's insistence on routine can come to dominate the life of the whole family.

The behavior is the child's attempt to introduce order into their chaotic world and this has to be remembered when working out the best way of managing the problem. It is necessary to arrange the child's life so that it has order and pattern. Some kind of repetitive behavior is inevitably present in a child with an autistic disorder and this has to be accepted. A firm line needs to be drawn when the routine or resistance to change reaches the point where it interferes with the life of the rest of the family and prevents the child from moving forward to more constructive activities.

The solution depends upon the nature of the routine. If the child insists on holding an object in their hand that is large and attracts adverse attention in public, or prevents other activities in which the hand would be used, or leads to other difficulties, the system of gradual reduction may be successful. One small girl insisted on holding a piece of photographic negative in her hand. Whenever the negative became creased or torn, which inevitably happened sooner or later, she screamed loud and long until a new piece was provided. Her parents decided to make the negatives a tiny bit smaller each day. This gradual change did not bother her. Eventually the stage was reached when the piece of negative was about one centimeter square. At this point a new problem emerged. The little girl held this in the center of the palm of her right hand with the tip of her middle finger. As soon as it became damp with perspiration, which occurred very frequently, she had a temper tantrum though she did not release her grip on the fragment of negative. Eventually her parents decided not to give her any more pieces and to ignore the screams. After a difficult day or two the child lost the last fragment and the routine disappeared.

Some objects cannot be cut down in size. One strategy that can be used is to allow the child to have the object at certain times and not at others. If for any reason the times when the object is to be allowed has to be reduced, this should be done gradually. Much determination is needed to start the process of time restriction but once established it becomes part of the child's routine. One ten-year-old girl wanted to carry a large dustpan and brush with her all the time. Her parents insisted that she leave it at home whenever she left the house. After a few protests she accepted the new routine of putting the dustpan and brush in one particular place and saying, "All ready for come back" when she went out.

There are other kinds of collecting that cannot be tackled by these methods. The case of the boy who wanted to hold empty detergent packets has already been mentioned in a previous chapter. He could find the packets in any house he was taken to visit and would run into a stranger's house if the door was open. If he found a packet with powder in it, he would empty it in the sink or on the floor. The only way his parents could deal with this was to prevent it altogether. They hid their own detergent packets, only visited friends and relations who understood and would do the same and kept a tight hold on the child's hand when out walking. They did not take him into any store that sold detergents. After a few weeks he had lost interest in this pursuit. If it is decided that some behavior has to be stopped and it cannot be done gradually, the policy of total prevention is the most likely to succeed, if it is possible to put this strategy into effect.

Some children involve other people in their routines. One child insisted that everyone in the family sit on the same chair at each meal. His temper tantrums if the pattern was disturbed made it impossible for the family to have guests for a meal. To overcome the problem the rest of the family decided to change their places at every meal, regardless of the tantrums. The child's protests became louder and longer for several days, then diminished over a few days and finally stopped completely.

Bedtime routines present particular problems. The children who have them may not settle to sleep until a complex sequence of actions involving the parents has been completed without error. It may be possible to diminish the routines by missing out a tiny step every few nights. Refusal to allow the routine at all is likely to lead to tantrums and refusal to settle down to sleep for some time. It is not possible to predict how long the protest might last. If the routine is not too taxing to carry out it is easiest to accept it, especially if the child then sleeps peacefully. It is worth taking a stand only if it is very long and complicated or if it seems to be growing in length and complexity.

Often parents who have had the courage to tackle a particular routine have found that once the problem has been overcome the child seems more aware of their parents in a positive way. The parents gain confidence in their ability to help their child, and the child finds that giving up a routine does not make the world fall to pieces. He or she has been helped to take a small step forward and the entire family gains from the experience.

It is one of the basic facts of autistic disorders that if one routine disappears another comes along to take its place. However, if one is overcome successfully by the parents, those that follow tend to present less of a problem. In theory it should be possible to deal with each routine as it occurs. In practice, most parents find that a compromise works well. Some of the habits comfort the child but do not cause any problems and these can be left alone. For example, it does not matter if a child likes to carry a particular small object in a pocket as long there is no tantrum if it is lost. Effort should be saved for tackling routines that do have adverse effects on the child or the family.

Once parents have made up their minds to discourage the unacceptable routines, it is helpful to deal with a new one that might be troublesome as soon as it appears. The task is easier in the early stages than once the routine is well established. A number of mothers take deliberate steps to vary household practices just a little every day so that the children become used to the idea of a certain amount of change. This may seem to contradict the rule that autistic children need order in their lives. The aim is to find a balance between too much rigidity on the one hand and too little structure on the other. How this is worked out depends on the individual child and the family concerned.

CHAPTER 11

Reducing Inappropriate Behavior

When a child with an autistic disorder begins to walk, the pattern of autistic behavior usually becomes obvious, whether or not there were signs during the first year or so. Parents have to begin the long process of helping their child to adapt to the family and the world. The problems they meet during the years of childhood are many and varied and each child has his or her own special difficulties, as well as those that are common to most autistic children. All I can do here is to write about some of the situations with which parents have to cope and to make some suggestions based on ideas that have proven helpful in practice.

It is easiest to consider ways of helping under two main headings. In this chapter I shall suggest ways of reducing inappropriate behavior. The following chapter will deal with methods for encouraging the development of skills. For each of these topics I shall give some general rules followed by practical examples of ways of helping the children.

These two chapters are concerned with autistic children, including those with severe autistic disorders and learning difficulties. The special problems and needs of adolescents and adults, and of those who are more-able will be considered in later chapters. However, the ideas in the discussion that follows are basic to all autistic disorders and have relevance for all ages and for all levels of ability.

General Principles

It is currently the fashion to refer to difficult behavior as "challenging." This term was chosen with the best of political intentions but the result has not always been that desired by those coining the phrase. It was meant to suggest that the behavior "challenged" the caregivers to find ways of helping the person concerned. Instead it is often thought of by those not in the field as behavior that is deliberately awkward and defiant, which excludes many of the types of behavior problems common in autistic disorders. The term "inappropriate" behavior seems to me to be both neutral and descriptive.

Until they know the reason, having a child with unusual and socially inappropriate behavior makes most parents feel that it is their fault even though the other children in the family may behave impeccably. These feelings are unjustified because the ordinary methods of bringing up children are based largely on the supposition that the child understands what you say, has some desire to please and has a growing awareness of the consequences of their actions. These do not work with children with autistic disorders.

In the first edition of this book, I discussed methods of rigid "behavior management" developed by psychologists and used with children with autistic disorders among others. These were based on theories of how people learn patterns of behavior through reward and punishment. At that time there was much interest in these ideas and hope that the methods would produce major improvements in behavior and level of ability. Over the years since then, the limitations of these methods, especially with regard to autistic children, have become apparent. Behavior management techniques do not help the children learn more than their built-in potential allows. The methods may sometimes, but by no means always, help to control behavior while they are being applied, but as soon as they cease the previous behavior returns. It was found that people with autistic disorders tend not to transfer any improvement in behavior or skills seen in one setting to other situations. Behavior management methods do not change the individual with an autistic disorder in any fundamental way—useful results, if any, are temporary.

Apart from the lack of permanent results, there have been two other major criticisms of these methods. First, in the early years some psychologists used harsh methods of discouraging inappropriate behavior that would now be considered to be abuse. In any case, many children with autistic disorders appear indifferent to physical punishment, have no notion of shame and tend to regard a punishment as an automatic part of a repetitive routine that is sought for rather than experienced as a deterrent. Second, the pioneers thought that the reasons for any behavior were irrelevant to its management and all one had to do was to apply the method strictly according to the rules. It is difficult to understand how anyone could have this view.

Although experience has shown the limitations of psychological methods of managing behavior, there are some general principles that parents and professionals have found useful, even if they do not solve all the problems. The first task is to sort out, if possible, the reasons for the inappropriate behavior. Here is a list of the most frequent reasons:

1. Interference with the usual daily routine or with the individual's own repetitive activities is perhaps the most frequent cause of difficult, inappropriate behavior. Alterations in tiny, trivial details may be enough to start a major temper tantrum.

2. Confusion and fear produced by unfamiliar events and situations.

3. Inability to understand explanations, reassurance or instructions.

4. Lack of knowledge of the social rules for behavior.

5. Inability to communicate needs and feelings in words or signs.

6. Over-sensitivity of the senses to such things as noise, bright lights, being touched, being in too close proximity to other people. Even smells can be the cause of intense distress and inappropriate behavior.

7. Specific fears (phobias) of harmless objects or situations.

8. Pressure to do tasks that are too difficult or that are disliked or that go on for too long.

9. Although other reasons are more common, parents and caregivers should consider the possibility that inappropriate behavior

is due to discomfort, pain or illness, especially if it is different in form or timing from the usual pattern.

Some general rules for coping with inappropriate behavior can also be listed although the way they are applied depends on the reasons for the behavior. The first seven of these are especially relevant for people with autistic disorders.

1. The first and most important rule has been emphasized. The environment and the daily routine must be structured, organized and predictable. The lack of ability to process information means that the person with an autistic disorder lives in a confusing and frighteningly unpredictable world. An organized environment and routine are vital in order to give them a feeling of order and stability.

2. Changes to the routine need to be planned, and if possible, introduced slowly. Ways have to be found to let the child or adult know in advance, as accurately as possible, what will happen. This is particularly important if there is to be a temporary or permanent change of caretakers for any reason. Attempts to change the child's own repetitive routines work best if carried out gradually, if this is possible.

3. Methods of communication have to be adapted to ensure that the child or adult understands what is wanted.

4. Ways need to be found to cope with aspects of the environment that cause distress, such as the level of noise, lighting that's too bright or the presence of something that is frightening for the child concerned.

5. Pressure to perform above the individual's level of ability must be avoided.

6. General health care and watchfulness for signs of injury or illness are important.

7. There is evidence that regular physical exercise tends to diminish aggressive behavior and stereotypies in people with autistic disorders as well as having beneficial effects on their health.

The last six rules come from general theories about learning.

8. Behavior that is rewarded is more likely to be repeated, while behavior that is not rewarded is less likely to be repeated. The dif-

ficulty is knowing what counts as a reward for people with autistic disorders. It can be something that others find uninteresting or even thoroughly unpleasant. Even the simple fact that an action has been carried out in a certain way is enough to begin a cycle of exact repetition.

9. With inappropriate behavior the best strategy is to prevent it occurring in the first place because it is so easy for people with autistic disorders to get into a repetitive cycle once they have started doing some action or sequence of actions.

10. If an inappropriate behavior cannot be prevented it should not be rewarded.

11. If at all possible, a different and more constructive activity should be provided and rewarded to replace the inappropriate behavior. The reward has to be relevant for the child concerned.

12. Timing is crucial. The response to behavior, whether it is to be encouraged or discouraged, should be timed so that it is quite clear that it is the behavior that produces the response. The poorer the understanding of language, the more important this is.

13. Inconsistency of response to inappropriate behavior, for example, sometimes ignoring, sometimes scolding and sometimes giving an ice cream to stop a temper tantrum, tends to make the behavior worse and certainly does not make it better.

These rules are not easy to follow in a family home, especially if there are other children, but they are worth attempting. Patience and perseverance are needed because results may not be seen for weeks, months or years. It helps a great deal to remain calm and avoid negative emotional reactions whatever the provocation. It cannot be said too often that the outward signs of anger are no help at all because many children and adults with autistic disorders find them interesting and rewarding and try to induce them again. It is helpful if parents work together and are consistent in the way they respond to inappropriate behavior.

The following are some examples of the way the rules can be applied in practice in response to particular aspects of behavior in autistic disorders.

Temper Tantrums and Aggression

Tantrums, which may be accompanied by biting, scratching or other aggressive acts towards the self or others, are common in children with autistic disorders. Methods of coping work best, and are in the best interests of the child and the whole family, if they take into account the reasons for the tantrums, though these may be difficult to discover. It is helpful to observe the situations in which tantrums occur to see if there is any pattern. Keeping notes is well worthwhile even if it is difficult to maintain consistently in the family situation.

When causes or precipitating factors are known, these should be eliminated or avoided if at all possible. If they cannot be avoided, at least the knowledge allows parents to anticipate and be ready to cope with the adverse reactions. When a tantrum or an aggressive act occurs, parents should respond in a calm, low-key way and should defuse the situation as soon as possible by, if necessary, removing the child from the place where the problem occurred and involving them in another activity. If a child tends to attack a sibling when upset this should be anticipated and prevented. Cooperation between all those caring for a child, planning in advance how to manage difficult behavior and consistency in response are particularly important in reducing physical aggression towards others.

The problems of tantrums in response to interference with repetitive routines have already been mentioned and ways of coping discussed.

Young children with autistic disorders often have tantrums simply because they want to be given something, such as a cookie or drink. Parents, understandably, tend to deal with the situation by giving the child what they want to soothe and quiet them because they know from bitter experience that the screams can go on for hours. Unfortunately, this is a good way to demonstrate the truth of one of the basic rules of learning theory—behavior that is rewarded tends to increase in frequency. In other words, the child finds out through practical experience that the quickest way to get anything they want is to scream, shout, stamp, kick, bite—in short to have a first-class temper tantrum. This behavior is one of the very limited options for a child with no useful spoken or signed language.

There are two aspects to changing this type of behavior. The first is to make sure that the children are never given the things they want while actually having a tantrum. This requires strong nerves and determination because the policy must be put into practice in public as well as at home. If a child has a tantrum because they have seen something they want in the street or in a store, the only solution may be to remove them from the scene rapidly, but with little fuss and as calmly as possible. In the home, some form of distraction may work, or holding the child while rocking and singing to them (if they like this) until the tantrum ceases, or ignoring the tantrum altogether are options. Experience shows what works best. If what the child wants is reasonable, it can be given when the tantrum stops but not before.

The second way of reducing temper tantrums used as demands is to encourage the development of more appropriate forms of communication, as discussed in Chapter 10. Even in children who have an adequate understanding of speech or signs, tantrums may occur if requests are refused. Many of them react very badly to the word "No." This is true of any young child but it is particularly evident in those with autistic disorders. It's a good idea to avoid the direct use of this word and of the sharp, negative tone of voice that goes with it. It is possible to use other calmly spoken words for refusing or deferring requests.

Screaming may be due to fear and distress produced by something that is in reality quite harmless. If this goes on for long, the child may lose all control and behave in exactly the same way as in a temper tantrum. When the cause is known, the child can be removed from the fear-provoking situation and comforted. Holding, cuddling and talking or singing in a soothing way until the child calms down is particularly appropriate for helping to reduce fear. The causes of the fear must be dealt with and some suggestions for this will be given below.

Some of the children resist and have tantrums in response to care procedures, especially hair washing, brushing, combing or cutting. The problem may be sensitivity to being touched, resistance to any interference, or it may be due to real fear. If the child dislikes being touched, it is important to be as gentle and reassuring as possible. If it is simply dislike of the interference, making the procedure part of the regular routine and calm, quiet persistence usually help the child to accept the procedures eventually. Distraction, such as playing a piece of music, may be helpful. If the child is obviously frightened, the suggestions given below in the section on special fears can be tried.

The Use of Medication

When tantrums and aggressive behavior are severe, frequent, prolonged and the cause cannot be identified and removed, medication may be considered as a last resort. The drugs used to influence behavior can be classified into groups with different types of effects. Some are intended to "tranquilize," that is, to calm and quiet by reducing responses to environmental stimuli. There are sub-groups in this category that achieve their effects through different kinds of biochemical actions.

In some people, disturbed behavior seems to be due to high anxiety. Sedatives or tranquilizers may help or a beta-blocker can be tried. The latter are drugs that are also used to treat high blood pressure. They act on the "autonomic" nervous system that controls heart rate, blood pressure, respiration and other systems that support life without needing conscious control. The beta-blockers are sometimes helpful in reducing anxiety and thereby produce calmer behavior, especially when disturbed behavior is accompanied by rapid pulse, sweating, large pupils and a general impression of agitation. Many beta-blockers, some more than others, can precipitate an attack of asthma in children or adults who are susceptible. This possibility has to be considered very carefully before a beta-blocker is prescribed.

Occasionally, episodes of disturbed behavior are related in some way to epilepsy and anti-epileptic medication proves helpful. In adolescents and adults, the cause of the disturbed behavior may be an underlying abnormality of mood, giving rise to depression or manic excitement, in which case drugs to treat depression or mania or alternations of these can be given. If other psychiatric conditions are present (see Chapter 12) these also may be treatable with appropriate medication.

It is difficult to predict the effect of any particular medication on people with autistic disorders. There are some general guidelines for deciding which drug to try, but it is always a matter of trial and error. Individuals may improve, there may be no effect, or there can be adverse effects, either severe side effects or a worsening of behavior. For these reasons, if medication is given the effects should be closely monitored.

There are some medications that may be given to people with autistic disorders to lessen overactive or disturbed behavior that make the skin sensitive to sunlight. This may cause swelling and a rash if the child spends any time in the sunshine. (In any case, the harmful effects for anyone to exposure to sunlight are now well-known.) Sunblock, clothing to cover arms and legs and shady hats are sensible measures. Parents should ask the doctor who prescribes any medication about light sensitivity and any other possible side-effects so that appropriate precautions can be taken.

Since medication for autistic disorders is not in any sense curative of the underlying impairments and acts only on aspects of behavior, it is preferable to use environmental and behavioral methods of treatment. This is particularly the case with children because their brains and nervous systems are still developing and the long-term effects of altering brain biochemistry in an immature central nervous system are not known. If medication is given, the dose should be as low as possible. If there is no effect or an adverse effect, the medication should be stopped, or if medically necessary, gradually withdrawn. Environmental and behavioral methods should always be used together with any medication.

Destructiveness and Interference with Others' Possessions

This is a serious problem for many parents. The children, especially when still at a low level of development, cannot play constructively so they often occupy themselves by examining the simple properties of the things around them. They soon discover that paper, including books and wallpaper, can be torn and that many hard things make a noise when hurled to the floor—and make an even more satisfying noise when they break. One small boy developed an unerring aim with his toy bricks and shattered all the light bulbs in his house. At a later stage the children develop enough to want to fit one object inside another. They often do not comprehend that large objects won't go into small, so they try force to achieve their aim, perhaps having a temper tantrum from frustration at the same time. The products of excretion are easily available so smearing the walls may be added to the rest of the damage. They may wander around the house, taking things out of cupboards and scattering them around the floor, leaving a trail of chaos for others to clean up.

While this stage lasts the same precautions have to be taken as one would for an active toddler. Things that are to be preserved, such as ornaments, or are dangerous, such as matches, have to be kept out of reach. Unbreakable crockery can be used and the best china put away. The kitchen may have to be locked if no one is in there to prevent accidents. Siblings, and parents as well, need somewhere where their special possessions are safe from the child. Precautions have to be taken to ensure that the child does not go uninvited into other people's houses.

Nighttime may be a special problem. The child's bedroom should be safe and easily cleaned. If the child tears the wallpaper one night when you are asleep there is no point in replacing it until this stage has passed. It is better to use a non-toxic washable paint that cannot be torn away.

Constant supervision is required at this stage of development. This can be exhausting if there is no relief. It may be possible for parents to share the burden to some extent or relatives may be able to help. Respite care on a regular basis, if the child accepts this without distress, can make things easier for the whole family.

The problems become less if and when the stage is reached at which more constructive activities can be introduced. If communication and understanding improve, the children can be taught that certain possessions are theirs but others are not and must not be touched. A set phrase to indicate ownership may help. One girl around seven, was taught to point to objects and say "That belongs to. . . ." She took delight in saying, "That belongs to Jenny" (her name), "That belongs to Daddy" and so on. This was made into a game in which a member of the family would touch something and say "That belongs to . . ." giving the wrong name. Jenny would then laugh with delight at the deliberate mistake and name the correct owner. She enjoyed this game and it gave her a better grasp of the concept of ownership.

Self-injury

Self-injurious behavior, varying from mild to severe, can occur in autistic disorders. The most severe and long-lasting self-injury occurs mostly in those with severe or profound levels of disability.

Minor forms of potentially self-injuring behavior are common in children with autistic disorders in association with temper tantrums. Biting the back of the hand and head banging are particularly frequent when the children are angry or upset. Coping with the tantrums helps to reduce this behavior.

Some children develop repetitive self-injurious behavior that is not confined to temper tantrums and continues for long periods of time. This can take many different forms, including biting, scratching and head banging. The effects vary in severity from trivial to extremely severe. Behavior such as regurgitating food, drinking excessive quantities of fluid, self-induced vomiting and poking fingers into body orifices can also be classed as self-injury.

Psychologists investigating self-injury suggest a number of interlinked causes that keep the behavior going even if they do not explain why it began in the first place. First, internal biological factors such as biochemical abnormalities may play a part in some cases. There are chemicals called opiates, resembling morphine, that occur naturally in the body. These reduce the feeling of pain and increase the feeling of well-being. Some of these chemicals are released in response to injury. One theory is that self-injury is a way of increasing the level of opiates in the body, thus increasing the feeling of well-being. Second, the sensations produced by the self-injury may be experienced as interesting, especially if biochemical factors reduce pain sensations. Third, environmental factors, especially the interaction with caregivers, are very important. For example, self-injury may be a way of obtaining a caretakers' attention or it may be a way of avoiding too high demands. Self-injurious behavior is most frequent in children who have little or no means of communication. In children with autistic disorders, the typical repetitiveness of the behavior pattern is another factor tending to make self-injury long lasting.

Psychologists concerned with treatment of self-injury emphasize the importance of finding, if possible, the function or functions of the behavior for the child or adult concerned. This is known as "functional analysis" and is done by careful observation and recording of the situations in which the behavior occurs. There are usually so many events during the course of any day that making records and selecting the crucial items is difficult. Computer technology is being developed to improve accuracy and make the task easier. With this information, the environment and the daily program can be planned to minimize the occurrence of self-injury. One promising approach, once the function of self-injury has been determined for an individual, is to teach other, more appropriate behavior to achieve the same goal or goals as the self-injury. In children with little or no means of communication, teaching ways of indicating their needs and wishes seems to be a way of preventing self-injury before it begins.

Protective clothing has been used to prevent serious injuries. This is best avoided if possible because the devices used tend to restrict movements so that engaging in other activities is difficult or impossible. Also, the child or adult may start to self-injure in order to have the protection put on. If it has to be used, the time for which the special clothing is worn should be kept as short as possible.

Various types of medication have also been tried. One class of drugs that do seem to help in some cases act against the natural opiate chemicals in the body. The opiate blockers reduce these levels so that the self-injury does cause pain. There are complicated ethical problems associated with this method. Even if protective clothing or medication is necessary as a short-term measure, they should be combined with functional analysis followed by behavioral methods based on the findings.

Chronic severe self-injury is one of the most distressing and difficult problems with which parents and caregivers have to cope. Advice should be sought as early as possible from psychologists with a special interest and experience in the field.

As with any type of behavior problem in autistic disorders, self-injury can be a sign of discomfort, pain or illness so this possibility should always be considered if the behavior newly appears or there is a marked change in the behavioral pattern. There are also a few congenital conditions in which self-injury is likely to occur, so medical examination is needed to see if any of these are present as well as the autistic disorder.

A review of recent advances in assessment and intervention has been written by Chris Oliver—see the reading list.

Restlessness and Hyperactivity

Most young children with autistic disorders are restless, often wandering around aimlessly. The great majority are not truly hyperactive and do not move about much more than most other children of the same age. They appear hyperactive because they have a short attention span and the consequences of their actions are undesirable from an adult point of view. They are either purposeless and randomly interfering or else are pursuing their repetitive routines regardless of anyone or anything else. This type of restless activity tends to be reduced if a structured program for each day is organized and more constructive activities encouraged (see Chapter 12).

There are a small number of children with autistic disorders who do have the additional problem of an attention deficit and hyperactive disorder. This combination of problems is particularly difficult to cope with in a family home. The same psychological approaches that help other children with autistic disorders are appropriate but may produce little result. In children of this kind, medication such as methylphenidate (Ritalin) may prove helpful in reducing activity level and improving attention while it is working. Although there can be undesirable side effects, they are unusual. If it is going to be effective, the results are seen immediately. If it does not work it should be discontinued without delay. Because it has been misused as a stimulant drug, this medication should be prescribed under the supervision of a physician specializing in behavioral disorders.

Socially Embarrassing Behavior

All young children are liable to cause embarrassment to their parents in public from time to time, providing many funny stories to be laughed at in retrospect. Children with autistic disorders do similar things, but they do them more often, they go on doing them for much longer and they do them with a total lack of inhibition.

With those whose comprehension of social rules is at a low level, anticipation of possible problems is essential. Shopping expeditions provide many opportunities for embarrassing behavior, such as knocking down a huge display of cans in a supermarket, or grabbing bars of chocolate at the check-out. The young children have no concept of barriers and will wander behind counters and into the back premises of shops quite unconcerned. Some of them run away at any opportunity, pursuing a straight course at considerable speed, ignoring all obstacles.

A small child may be willing to sit in the supermarket basket or stay in a stroller, but they soon grow too big for these measures. The child can be encouraged to hold a basket and eventually to push the stroller. A consistent, patient approach and constant repetition are needed to develop positive behavior in stores. When an action has to be prevented, it is better to give an instruction for alternative behavior than to say "No" or "Don't do that." For example, a calm but firm command to "Hold my hand" combined with taking the child's hand can forestall the act of grabbing something from the shelves.

Visits to stores should, if at all possible, be planned so that they are short and scheduled at times when few people are around until the child is more able to cooperate. It is easier to cope with shopping and to try to teach appropriate behavior if two adults are involved. Close supervision and the prevention of any inappropriate behavior can be the task of one while the other adult shops. Among other advantages, one adult can take the child out of the store to avoid a long line at the check-out stand, the point at which any child, let alone one with an autistic disorder, may behave inappropriately.

Particular social problems arise with those who can talk well. The children's habit of echoing words and phrases they have heard in the past can lead to unfortunate consequences. Parents have to be especially careful of the things they say in front of their child if they do not want them repeated in an exact copy of their accents and tone of voice. Swear words are particularly easy to learn because the emphasis and intensity usually accompanying them catch the attention even of a child with little speech and poor comprehension. Naive remarks about other people, made in a loud voice, have to be discouraged.

The older children's lack of appreciation of social taboos often leads to problems. Removing clothes or urinating in public may be done in all innocence by an adolescent or young adult. Parents and teachers have to lay down a series of rules in an attempt to forestall or prevent a repetition of such incidents. The trouble is that no one can think of everything that might happen and life seems too short to teach the correct response in every imaginable situation, let alone the unimaginable ones that seem to crop up just as often. One can only do what one can and hope for the best. Once a rule is learned, an autistic child tends to keep it under all circumstances. This leads to problems too, as with the child who learned that one must always urinate in a lavatory and then suffered intense discomfort on a long drive in the countryside because he could not be persuaded to break the rule in this special situation. It is important to remember to show pleasure and appreciation when an outing has passed without a mishap.

Carol Gray has developed a method of encouraging appropriate social behavior through "social stories," written in words and pictures for the individual child, incorporating information and tactfully phrased instructions geared to their level of understanding and their special interests. This is a way of translating social rules into visible form and can be helpful for children with the ability to understand the simple stories. The method would be applicable to adults as well as children. Carol Gray's materials can be incorporated into an intervention plan by professionals who work with autistic children. The availability of professionals who have been specifically trained in social stories is relatively low and will vary from area to area. Materials can be purchased through Future Horizons, Inc., 800-489-0727; www.futurehorizons-autism.com.

The consequences of a child's inappropriate behavior can be more serious for the parents than simple embarrassment. Occasionally, a child with an autistic disorder has repetitive behavior or speech that appears to have a sexual content. They can hear things from other children and repeat them in all innocence. One child, for example, sat through a sex education class at school and then constantly repeated the half-understood words and phrases regardless of where she was. This led to an investigation of possible sexual abuse, to the distress of the parents. In other cases, parents have been suspected of physical abuse because their child frequently shouts out angry, scolding words.

It is, of course, possible for children with autistic disorders to be abused in all kinds of ways, but a high level of knowledge and experience of autistic conditions is required to assess each situation and to reach a proper conclusion. The content of repetitive speech or behavior on their own is a very poor guide to the home life of the child. Why the children latch on to obscenities and angry words and tones of voice no one knows. It is a fact that many do this once they have started school and have met other children with colorful vocabularies. In this situation it is helpful to both the parents and the professionals involved to seek advice from someone with specialized experience in the field of autistic disorders.

Special Fears

Some of the children are always tense and fearful and many develop fears of harmless things at some time or other. It is usually difficult to know the origin of the fears, but sometimes it is possible to trace them back to their beginnings. One little girl had a pair of new shoes that were uncomfortable because they rubbed her heels. From then on she screamed and refused to walk if shoes were put on her feet. After a time, she began to scream even at the sight of her shoes or slippers. A small boy put his finger into a bath of water that was a little too hot and could not be persuaded to enter the bath for years after that, although he was quite happy to sit in the large kitchen sink. Children who are developing normally may have experiences that alarm them when they are small, but usually they can communicate their fears to their parents and accept verbal reassurance and explanation. Children with autistic disorders have no way of asking for help and unexpected or distressing events tend to confirm their fears of the world and their dislike of any change.

The behavior that was first caused by fear may continue as a routine habit long after the fear has gone. In this case it can be dealt with in the same way as other routines. Before this stage is reached the problem is more difficult to solve because the child's terror is so obvious and parents feel acute distress if they try to force the child into such frightening situations.

The most helpful approach is very gradual exposure to the frightening situation, known in psychological jargon as "desensitization." It works best if each exposure is accompanied by something the child does enjoy. For example, the little girl who would not wear shoes was helped in the following way. At the time she loved to eat boiled eggs. When she had her egg for snack, a pair of slippers in her favorite color was placed beside her while she was eating and taken away before she had finished. Without the egg the slippers produced screams, but with the egg they were accepted calmly. The time with the slippers was lengthened until the stage was reached when they could be put on her feet while she was eating. The time with slippers on was again lengthened until she wore them cheerfully all through her snack. After this, her outdoor shoes were tried and these produced no fearful reaction. She wore them without any fuss and from then on they were put on in the morning in the usual way. The fear never recurred and buying new shoes is now looked forward to as a pleasant occasion.

It is not always possible to carry out this kind of plan. Chocolates were tried for James, the little boy who was afraid of the bathtub, but the fear was too strong to be soothed by the candy. It is interesting that this problem was eventually overcome in a different and unexpected way. Maria, an au pair living with the family who was good with children, popped him into a bath on the first day she arrived, unaware of his fear. His astonished mother heard happy giggles and splashes and found her child enjoying his first bath in years as if he had one every day. Encouraged by her success, Maria persuaded James to use the bathroom, of which he had previously been afraid. In this case, it seems that the child was helped by the fact that Maria was not anticipating fear, whereas his parents had grown accustomed to it. They also learned from the experience and were much more confident and successful in dealing with other, similar problems that occurred after this incident. It is interesting that Maria, who arrived knowing hardly any English, developed a close rapport with James because, as she explained, they both had a language problem and both were, so to speak, strangers in a strange land.

Another approach to fear of having a bath can be tried with children who are worried about the water, not the bathtub itself. The child is placed in the empty bath, perhaps in a swim suit if swimming is enjoyed, with some favorite waterproof toys. After a few sessions of this, a small amount of water is introduced. If this is accepted, then the amount of water is gradually increased day by day until the child accepts enough for a bath. The important point about desensitization is that each step should cause no anxiety. Care has to be taken to ensure that the triggers for fear are identified and that the whole sequence of steps is organized to deal with these. For example, if undressing in the bathroom sets off a panic attack, the plan would have to be modified to take account of this. If it is the sound of the water entering or leaving the bath, the problem might be solved if the tub is always filled and emptied when the child is well out of earshot.

As mentioned previously, some of the children are terrified of hair care, especially having their hair cut. This is a difficult problem to deal with. Occasionally a child is so frightened that the hair is not cut for years, or attempts are made to cut it while the child is asleep. Taking a child to a hairdressing salon can be a nightmare so some parents arrange for a hairdresser to come to their home. Techniques of distraction can be tried but are less likely to succeed where there is great fear. One variation of the distraction method is to produce something, such as a particular object, toy or food that the child likes very much, only during hair cutting if the child is cooperative. It can also happen that a child accepts hair cutting without protest if accompanied by someone other than his or her parents, so this is worth trying, perhaps with the help of someone from the child's school.

Some families have dealt with their child's fear of dogs by buying a small puppy. This usually, though not always, works well. It is wise to choose a dog from a reputable breeder and of a type that is likely to be placid and good with children when grown up. This solution is not recommended unless the parents are fond of dogs and know exactly what the care of a pet entails. They should also arrange in advance a possible alternative home for the puppy in case the child's fear of dogs does not improve.

Children with autistic disorders can develop a whole range of fears because of their sensitivity to loud noises, bright lights or other sensations. This may lie behind fears of, for example, airplanes, trains, motor-bikes, barking dogs and photographers' flashes, or putting on clothes made of rough material. They find these stimuli painful and are not making a fuss about nothing. Calm reassurance and distraction of the child's attention may help if the sensitivity is not too severe. If it causes too much distress, especially if it interferes with everyday activities, gradual desensitization can be very effective. Some clinical psychologists are particularly interested in these types of problems and parents can seek their help in working out a program.

It can happen that a child overcomes a fear through a chance event. A girl liked to jump up and down in the water at the ocean but would scream if anyone tried to hold her so that her feet did not touch the bottom. One day she accidentally tripped and lost her footing but found that she was able to float with her special arm floats and swimming ring. From that moment she was utterly without fear of the ocean, and in fact, became rather over confident for her own safety. Parents may be tempted to try the method of instant exposure to a feared situation, but it can fail and intensify the fear. The method of gradual desensitization is much safer and surer.

Lack of Fear of Real Dangers

This is the opposite side of the picture to the children's special fears, but can be equally worrying. Total lack of road sense is almost universal in autistic children. The children who like climbing tend to have at least one heart-stopping feat to their credit, such as walking along a narrow ledge on the roof or hanging out of the window practically by their toes. They are usually so sure-footed that no harm results, but there have been a very few instances in which children have been injured or killed because they were oblivious of real danger.

Parents have to be aware of this. They can teach the rules for crossing the road, avoiding fires, electricity and gas, and warn of other common dangers, but even the brightest of autistic children will learn these by rote and may not apply them to a new situation. All possible sources of danger both inside and outside the house have to be considered and proper precautions organized.

Stereotyped Movements

The repetitive bodily movements that are so common in children with autistic disorders are not disruptive for other people but they do look strange and attract attention and criticism in public, especially in an older child or adult.

The movements tend to diminish or cease when the child is involved in a more constructive activity, especially if this requires movements that are incompatible with the stereotypies. This is why they are much less in evidence in a well-run classroom at school than they are in the playground during unstructured break times. When out in public, one useful strategy for parents is to give the child something to carry, such as a shopping bag or the supermarket basket to push. Holding hands with someone else also helps, if the child will accept this.

It is not possible or desirable to try to suppress the child's movements completely. Attempts to do so leads to a build-up of tension and distress. Some very able adults have described how they feel the need to engage in their stereotyped movements during some time each day. The eventual aim is to diminish or stop them in public or when they interfere with other activities but allow them in privacy at specific times. This aim can be achieved for many people with autistic disorders, but for those with the most severe disabilities it may not be possible to make much difference to their stereotypies.

Problems with Eating

Eating problems are common in the early years. At least two different factors may be involved in feeding problems and food fads. First, some children with autistic disorders have trouble controlling the movements of the muscles involved in chewing and swallowing. They are difficult to wean because they do not know how to cope with lumpy food. It is interesting to note that children born with severe visual disabilities combined with severe hearing impairments also often reject lumpy food. Food that needs chewing has to be introduced slowly so that the child can practice without being frightened by lumps that are too big or hard to manage. One mother found that she had to teach her son to chew by moving his lower jaw with her hands to give him an idea of the movements required. Speech therapists have developed a series of exercises designed to help children who have trouble in coordinating tongue and mouth movements. These include blowing bubbles, blowing pieces of cotton wool and retrieving sweet food placed on the lips outside the mouth by using the tip of the tongue.

The second major reason for feeding problems arises from the children's resistance to change and their tendency to cling to special routines. Minor eating problems of this type can be dealt with by providing a good mixed diet, giving food only at mealtimes and adopting an attitude of casual indifference to how much is eaten. If the child takes in adequate quantities of essential nutrients and fluid it does not matter if they refuse certain kinds of food, or eat only one meal a day. In this situation, there is no need for a mother to cook special food for the child because the rest of the family likes carrots and the child with autism never touches them. Children can miss a meal occasionally without coming to any harm and may be more likely to come around to trying something new if they are hungry and know they will get nothing else.

A number of the children go through phases in which their diet is restricted to a very few foods, for example, hamburgers and fries, or cereals and bread and butter cut into pieces of a precise size and shape. Usually, the foods they will eat are those that do not require lengthy chewing. Parents sometimes try to change the child's eating routine by allowing them to miss one or two meals in the hope that hunger will persuade them to eat additional types of food. Occasionally this works, but more often these children appear indifferent to hunger and can last without food much longer than the parents are prepared to withhold meals. Providing that autistic children will eat some things, it is surprising how active and healthy almost all of them remain on the diets they choose.

It is important to remain outwardly calm and to show no anxiety about meals. This is a reasonable attitude considering how little the children's peculiar diets affect their health or even their weight. One tactic that sometimes helps is to provide the food the child will eat but to add a tiny quantity of some other food, preferably something that is not noticeably different in appearance. If this is accepted, the quantity can be increased gradually and then other foods added. However, some children notice the added food at once and refuse to eat any of the meal so this method will not work for them. Restricted diets are usually a passing phase, though they can last for years. The problem may disappear when the child starts school and has school meals, although some retain their special diet at home while eating a wide range of foods at school and elsewhere.

Some of the children will not eat with others but may eat if given meals on their own. Some will take food left for them if they are allowed to eat while moving around. For some, the texture of the food is the crucial factor such as the child who will eat only uncooked, crunchy vegetables and fruit. The immediate problem of eating sufficient food can be solved by observing what, where and when the child will eat and fitting it in with these idiosyncrasies. The longer-term problem of encouraging more conventional eating patterns has to be approached gradually and may need an individualized program designed by a psychologist with experience in this field.

Most of the children will drink fluids even if they eat only a few foods. If needed, protein and vitamin supplements can be given in flavored liquids.

There have been a very few cases of children who will eat nothing at all or who eat so little that their health is at risk. In such cases, medical and psychological help is required. There are a few centers in hospitals that have a special interest in feeding problems where advice on treatment can be obtained; for instance the Children's Hospital in Richmond, Virginia, has a Pediatric Feeding Disorders Program that treats children age birth to 21 who present different underlying conditions such as autism. If your child has a severe feeding problem, contact hospitals in your area to determine the nearest specialty program.

If a feeding problem starts in a child who has previously eaten reasonably well the parents should make sure that the child does not have some physical illness, such as a fever or a painful mouth or throat that has caused the loss of appetite.

Problems with Sleeping

Some children with autistic disorders sleep well but others are poor sleepers. They may resist going to bed, lie awake once they are in bed, wake in the night and laugh, sing, and if they have speech, talk to themselves, wander around the house or get into their parents' bed, wake very early and refuse to go back to sleep, or any combination of the above. Some sleep very little and some seem never to adjust to the usual cycle of waking and sleeping.

Medication for inducing sleep may be helpful but it should be used only as a temporary measure. Some children are resistant and need a larger than usual dose, which should only be given on medical advice. For some, medication has the opposite effect than intended and makes the child more active and irritable. It is very possible that new drugs with more specific effects on the physiology of sleeping will become available so it is worthwhile for parents to ask from time to time about the latest developments in this field.

A behavioral approach devised by specialist psychologists may work well. Briefly, the aim is to ensure that the child remains in bed, or at least in the bedroom, during the night. The child is put to bed at a reasonable time and then whenever he or she gets up and leaves the bedroom, the parent returns the child to bed without any fuss, remaining with the child for as short a time as possible. Similarly, if the child wakes in distress and cries or screams, the parent should use any soothing tactics that work in the bedroom and not take the child downstairs or into the parents' own bed. If the child will not sleep without a parent in the room the plan is for the parent to move a little farther away from the child each night or every few nights until finally she or he is outside the room. The process may take a long time, but if successful, the effort is worthwhile. It helps if the parents take turns to be on night duty so that each has some sleep.

Unfortunately there is no guarantee of success. These problems tend to be most severe in the pre-school years and may improve spontaneously once the child goes to school each day. Regular physical exercise may also help.

Quiet, Withdrawn Children

So far I have described the behavior of the children with autistic disorders who are active and react to their disabilities with a kind of angry determination. There are other children, a small minority, who respond in a different way. They are quiet and withdrawn, tending to isolate themselves from the world rather than hitting their heads against it in rage and frustration. They may be un-childlike in their neatness and cleanliness because they never explore their environment and have no interest in mud, sand or water. In contrast to the active child who climbs to the top shelf of the cupboard to reach forbidden objects and undoes locks in a way that Houdini would have envied, the passive children may do nothing for themselves. They give the impression that their hands lack the strength even to lift a spoon to their mouths, or to handle a toy that is placed in front of them.

This kind of child is less difficult to live with than those who are full of energy, but they tend to be even more detached and indifferent to affection. The book *The Siege*, by Clara Claiborne Park, a parent of a child of this kind, gives an excellent and moving description of the way in which she helped her daughter. She also gives detailed advice that other parents can follow. Despite her remoteness as a small child, Clara's daughter gradually emerged from this withdrawn state and developed a range of abilities, including a remarkable skill with numbers.

Children of this kind, because they are quiet and gentle, may not be recognized as having a disorder in the autistic continuum and may be expected to fit into mainstream education with little or no special provision. At adolescence some become disturbed and difficult, a stark contrast to their amiability in childhood. The nature of their problems then becomes much more obvious. If the diagnosis is made when the child is young, the possibility of problems in adolescence can be anticipated and to some extent avoided by providing appropriate education and help from early childhood.

CHAPTER 12

Teaching Basic Skills

In the past many children with autistic disorders were excluded from the educational system. Some parents undertook the task of teaching schoolwork to their own children. Now, autistic children can attend school and parents do not have to take on the dual role. However, learning the basic skills of life begins in the home. Parents of children with autistic disorders often have a hard time trying to help them develop these skills. Some suggestions based on practical experience will, I hope, be of help.

General Principles

The suggestions are only of use if they are applied with a full understanding of the level and pattern of abilities and disabilities of each individual child. A good level of skill in one area does not mean an equally good level in another. Pressing someone with an autistic disorder to attempt a task beyond their ability is a sure way to induce inappropriate behavior. On the other hand, no progress is made unless new things are tried. Parents and teachers have to tread a narrow line between too many demands and too few. Parents develop a deep knowledge of their own child while teachers develop a broad knowledge of many children. Cooperation between the two is the ideal. A number of rules based on theories of how people learn are particularly relevant to teaching new skills. These are as follows —the first two were also mentioned in Chapter 11:

1. Behavior that is rewarded is more likely to be repeated than behavior that is not rewarded. As has already been emphasized, the

problem is to find what acts as a reward for any individual child with an autistic disorder. Music, pleasant sensory stimuli and social attention may be successful if the child enjoys them. Objects, activities or special interests that are part of the child's repetitive routines can be very effective as incentives. Experience has shown that they can be used without leading to other problems.

2. Timing of the reward is important so that the child connects it with the behavior.

3. New skills are learned more easily if they are broken down into small, easy steps. Children with autistic disorders are especially liable to be upset by failure so making sure that the child can succeed at each small stage is important.

4. With some tasks it is best to begin with the last step, then the next to last, and so on, so that the child is aware of completing a task successfully. This is called "backward chaining." (Examples will be given later.)

5. Prompts that help the child to succeed should be given at first and then gradually made less obvious ("faded") as the child learns the task and until prompts are no longer needed.

6. When trying to encourage the development of a new skill or change a behavior pattern, the child should be asked to perform the new activity for a very brief time at first and allowed to stop before they become bored and restless—or worse, have a temper tantrum. The time can be extended very gradually.

7. The tendency to repetition of actions previously performed, despite the many problems associated with it, can be used in teaching the child. The difficulty lies in finding ways to encourage the performance of a new action in the first place.

The Pattern of Skill Development

The children often make very slow progress, or none at all for months or years. This is disappointing and frustrating for parents. However, children with autistic disorders typically have an unusual type of "learning curve." This means that instead of making steady progress, however slow, they tend to learn something then stay at this point for a long time—they reach a "plateau." Then when everyone has given up hope, they suddenly take a step forward. Sometimes they appear to learn something without preliminary practice. There are many examples, such as the boy of nine who tied his own shoelaces one day after his mother had tied them for him every morning up to that time. A girl refused to try to ride a bicycle, then, at age 12, she took her bike out of the garage and rode it competently around the garden. Sometimes there is an obvious reason for the change but often no explanation can be found. The special skills mentioned in Chapter 3, such as drawing, numerical or calendar calculations, that are found in perhaps one in ten children with autistic disorders, usually emerge more or less fully formed without previous practice.

Occasionally a child will perform a new skill once only and it may be many years before they try again. It is realistic to expect a slow rate of progress on a different time scale from that of most children. Most, however, do make at least some progress in acquisition of skills and this can continue into adult life.

Encouraging Cooperation

Children with autistic disorders have no innate desire to please anyone else or to accept authority. The language difficulties limit comprehension of instructions and lead to confusion about what is required. In addition, many children with autistic disorders are extremely distressed by any failure and hate to be corrected if they make an error.

It is very easy to overestimate how much the children understand what is said to them. Those with little or no speech rely on visual clues rather than the words they hear. The children who say a great deal but are using the store of words in their rote memory appear to understand far more than they really do. One of the effects of poor understanding is that the child may pick up and respond to only one or two words in a sentence. The words that mean something to them are usually the nouns and some verbs specifying actions. Other words that are crucial to the meaning of an instruction may be incomprehensible and therefore ignored. For many children with poor understanding, the word "Don't" may be an irrelevant noise, so the instruction "Don't touch the oven" may be misinterpreted as "Touch oven," with disastrous consequences. This is one of the reasons why the children may appear to choose to act in negative ways. Parents and anyone living or working with a child or adult with an autistic disorder always need to be aware of the limits of their understanding and to adjust the words they use accordingly. Positive instructions, for example, are simpler and easier to understand than those given in negative terms.

Methods of teaching and ways of communicating have to be tailored to the child's level of understanding and ability to perform any skill. If the child's developmental level is too low for learning a particular task, the child is likely to react negatively if attempts to teach that skill are continued. It is important to begin at a low level, well within the child's capacity, so that they are rewarded by success. The rate at which difficulty is increased has to be determined according to the child's progress. If, after trying to teach a child, it becomes obvious that he or she is not ready for that particular task, it should be left for a while and then tried later. It requires considerable insight and judgement to decide at any particular stage if increased pressure will help a child to succeed, or if it will intensify confusion and anxiety. The patchiness of the profile of skills that is so common in autistic conditions makes it difficult to assess ability in any one area.

There is no easy answer to this problem and parents and teachers have to decide the best course of action in light of their knowledge of and feeling for the child and their past experience. It helps to remain calm, confident and reassuring because the children are sensitive to the emotions of people who are involved with them. If it is felt the child can succeed, the parent or teacher must be firm and show that he/she has to try, but they must not lose their temper if the child fails. If the parent or teacher is mistaken they must accept defeat with good grace and not blame the child.

In the pre-school years, autistic children may show no reaction when spoken to and may even ignore the sound of their own name.

If this is the case, it helps to link it deliberately to situations that are enjoyed, such as mealtimes, drinks and snacks, getting ready for an outing, physical play. The child's name can be introduced into favorite songs, especially when holding and cuddling the child. It is also sensible not to use the child's name a great deal in situations where the child is not required to respond. Parents and teachers should, for instance, avoid discussing a child in their presence because, apart from other objections, this allows them to fall back into the habit of hearing their name spoken while ignoring it.

Dislike of physical contact, which usually affects gentle touch rather than hugging and rough-and-tumble play, can make a child even less willing to cooperate. Suggestions for reducing this have been given in Chapter 10.

Some children with autistic disorders, and adults too, hardly ever choose to sit down even when engaged in activities such as eating, watching videos or listening to music. Many never learn to sit for very long but can be encouraged to sit for meals if they are only allowed food while sitting down at the table. As with most attempts to change behavior, the gradual approach is the best. At first, the child should be expected to sit only while eating. If this works well, it may be possible to slowly increase the time at table. This approach is only relevant for the children who positively enjoy their food and will eat when sitting down.

If activities such as playing with musical or constructional toys, looking at picture books, making jigsaw puzzles, drawing and painting are enjoyed, the materials can be produced only when the child is sitting down. It is easier for a child to stay sitting if an adult sits with them and helps them to engage in the activities. The session should finish before the child becomes restless and can be followed by something more active. The time will be short at first but can be extended gradually.

It is difficult for children whose speech is mainly echolalia to express a preference if asked to choose between two or more items. In response to the question, "Do you want an apple or an orange?" the child may repeat the whole sentence, or else echo the last word ("orange") even if it was the apple that was preferred. It is easier for them to make a choice if they can see the alternatives and touch the one they want. There is then the opportunity for the parent to say, for example, "Apple please" while giving the apple, so that the child will echo this, and eventually, use the construction appropriately.

Many young autistic children develop the habit of saying "No" automatically when asked if they want something. It is part of ordinary social interaction to ask, for example, "Do you want some toast?, Do you want juice?, Do you want to go for a walk?" At the stage when the child answers in the negative, even if they do want whatever is offered, it is best to make the decision for the child without asking. This may appear to be depriving the child of choice. The reality is that they deprive themselves as a result of their social and language impairments. The way to ensure that the wishes of the child are taken into account is for parents or caregivers to observe the reactions to whatever is chosen for them and to note them for future action.

When a skill is learned the child may repeat it again and again until its performance seems meaningless and may resist any attempt to move on to another task. The methods of dealing with repetitive routines described in Chapter 10 are helpful in this situation.

Even if all the rules for encouraging interest in developing skills are followed, many of the children vary markedly in their cooperativeness from one time to another. Parents often notice that their children seem to have good days and bad days. Sometimes they are more alert, more interested in the world and more willing to learn. At other times, perhaps even the next day, they are withdrawn, irritable and refuse to cooperate. Occasionally parents notice that their child's appearance is subtly different on the bad days, perhaps looking pale with dark circles round the eyes. The reasons for these variations are unknown but it is possible that they are due to cyclical physical changes. On a day when a child is clearly functioning less well than usual it is best not to press them to do things they find difficult.

Toilet Training

Some autistic children are toilet trained without any difficulty and some become clean and dry at an unusually early age. Others are late in learning and may resist any attempt to train them. The training methods that are used with other children may be successful with those who have autistic disorders but they require a high degree of patience and persistence. The general rule is not to make any fuss about the children's mistakes, but to put them on the potty or toilet regularly, especially at the times when they are most likely to need to empty their bowels or bladder. These times are usually on waking after a dry night or daytime nap, after meals and after drinks given between meals. Each child has to be observed carefully so that the time between eating or drinking and emptying bowels or bladder can be worked out fairly accurately. If successful the child should be given lots of praise and attention, or some other suitable reward. If nothing happens no emotion should be shown.

The trouble is that methods that work with other children are often of no use at all with children with autistic disorders. Some of them seem to dislike or even fear the potty or toilet. It is worthwhile trying to find out if they feel uncomfortable or insecure, and if so, for what reason. Small potty-chairs can be bought that are stable and comfortable. An adult-size toilet may be too high off the ground for a small child so something to place his feet on will help. A very cold seat will be enough to worry some children. The flushing of the toilet may terrify some, though it can fascinate others.

Resistance to change in an established routine is one of the reasons for delay in toilet training. There are a number of children who will wet or soil or both only when wearing a diaper. They have excellent bowel and bladder control because they can remain clean and dry for hours until a diaper is put on them. As babies they learned to associate bowel and bladder function with wearing a diaper and cling to this routine after infancy has passed. One approach that may work is to try to change the routine gradually by putting a diaper on the child followed immediately by sitting them on the potty or toilet. If the child accepts this, the diaper could be put on more loosely, then just draped over the potty or toilet seat, then gradually reduced in size until it is no longer needed.

Self-care

This includes dressing, using a knife, fork and spoon, washing, brushing and combing hair, cleaning teeth and all the other necessities of daily living. Children who are not disabled try to imitate these activities, which they see performed by other members of the family. When they are strong enough and coordinated enough, they begin to cooperate in the care given by their parents and soon want to take over these functions for themselves. They want to try washing, dressing and feeding themselves even if they make a mess in the process. Children with autistic disorders, on the other hand, may go through a phase, around one or two years of age, of actively resisting attempts to wash and dress them. Every item of daily care may precipitate a tantrum at this stage. Later on they tend to accept all these attentions passively. Having been cared for by others from birth, they resist any change in the daily program especially if some effort is demanded of them.

Young children with autistic disorders usually do not learn practical skills by being told how, nor by being shown how. However, they may learn by direct experience. If a child is physically guided through the pattern of movements necessary for a particular skill the chances are they will eventually be able to follow the pattern on their own. For example, a mother taught her little boy to fasten buttons as follows. She chose a garment with large buttons and easy buttonholes on the front. She stood behind the child and held his hands firmly, but not too tightly, so that she could guide them through the movements necessary for fastening the buttons. At first his fingers felt limp and his mother had to do all the work. After about a week, she began to feel some tension in his hands. Little by little he followed her movements until in the end he was fastening the buttons by himself. This type of teaching can be adapted for other self-care tasks as well as many other kinds of physical activities.

It is also helpful to break tasks down into simple steps. It is often best to teach the last step first and work backwards so the child is always the one to finish the job—the process known as "backward chaining." For example, when learning to put on socks, the child is first taught to pull them up after the foot and heel are in place. When this is mastered, the next step is to pull the sock over the heel and so on.

Dressing is a special problem because it involves putting things on the right way out, the right way around and in the right sequence. If you consider all the operations involved in putting on a pullover with the seams inside and the V-neck in front, you can see that it is a most complicated activity. Even when a child is able to put clothes on they may still need to be taught how to put them on in the right order and the right way around. To start with, it will be necessary to place the clothes in front of the child in the correct order and arranged so that they will end up in the correct position and to give a guiding hand when necessary. Some children are helped by labels that indicate the inside and back of garments.

One difficulty is that autistic children do not have much conception of a finished result. They do not put the final touches to dressing, such as tucking a shirt inside pants, or pulling up the socks neatly. Hair tends to be brushed the requisite number of times without regard to the actual style in which it is supposed to be worn and without thinking about the back, which cannot be seen in a mirror. Face and hands may be washed with vigor, but without removing streaks of dirt on areas left untouched by the operation. They are often unaware of which clothes are suitable for the prevailing weather and will put on thick underclothes in the summer, or light T-shirts in the winter. Supervision and tactful assistance or verbal reminders are necessary. Such help should be given gently and pleasantly without any hint of criticism or nagging.

An interest in clothes and general appearance is a good thing to encourage. It is worthwhile taking extra trouble to dress the children so that they look as neat and attractive as possible. This is a help towards being accepted socially and also provides a reason for people to make nice remarks to the child. As they grow older, the children may begin to take some interest in their clothes and enjoy expeditions to buy new ones. This is a happy contrast to the early years when many autistic children furiously resist any attempt to try on clothes in stores.

The children should be encouraged to feed themselves even if they are messy eaters. They may have to use only a spoon and fork for a long time. Some of them find problems in coordinating a knife and fork for cutting food and may manage better if allowed to eat pre-cut food with a fork alone.

Helping in the Home

Children with disabilities are dependent for so long and need so much special care that they tend to become passive members of their families. It is better for them if they have some positive role to play, however limited this may be. Setting the table is one task that many can achieve and can be taught by physically guiding the child through the movements. Carrying out the task provides the opportunity for learning the names of the implements, counting the places to be set and naming each person who will take part in the meal.

Clearing the table, taking out the trash, carrying a small shopping bag, pushing a basket in a supermarket, wheeling a small wheelbarrow in the garden are other examples of tasks that even young or very disabled children can take part in. Jobs that are quick to perform are best to start with. It is more difficult to persuade the children to persist at an endless task like clearing leaves from the lawn. They cannot understand the purpose and soon wander away. When they are older they may become better at such tasks.

If a task involves a sequence of operations, many of the children tend to forget the steps involved. One little girl of seven was helping in the garden by taking a basket full of weeds to the compost pile. She set off down the long garden path, then after a few yards she stopped and looked puzzled. Her father repeated the instructions, her face cleared and she set off again, only to stop once more. She finally reached the destination and disposed of the weeds, but had to have the separate instructions repeated four times altogether. After a while she had the whole task clear in her mind and could carry it out unaided.

Children who can say some words may be able to learn to take simple messages. These should at first relate to something that the child likes, such as letting someone know that a meal is ready. If the child enjoys eating or drinking, they are likely to be willing to take such a message when they make a connection with the fact that they also will have the meal. Depending on the child's level of ability, teaching may require a number of steps. In this example, the first step is to practice saying the phrase, "Lunch is ready, Mary." Then the child can be led to Mary (who is primed in advance) and prompted by a whisper to say the words, "Lunch is ready, Mary." Mary then shows great pleasure, thanks the child and all go to have lunch. Gradually the prompt should be faded, then the child taken only part of the way until they can take the message on their own.

One problem in teaching a child with an autistic disorder to carry messages is their lack of understanding that words have to be heard by the recipient for them to have any effect. They tend to assume that speaking the words is sufficient regardless of where the other person is at the time. This is all part of their incomprehension of the purposes and methods of communication. This has to be taken into account when teaching.

Toys and Games

The impairment of imagination severely limits the range of toys and games that children with autistic disorders can make use of and enjoy. They tend to prefer toys that involve visuo-spatial skills such as shape and color-matching, jigsaw puzzles or constructional materials. There is now a wide range of mechanical and electrical equipment for children that is attractive to many children with autistic disorders, especially those who are more able. Computers and computer games are particularly fascinating, even to some who have few skills in other areas. Computer technology is being applied to the educational and leisure needs of children with disabilities and it is well worth keeping up with the latest advances. The disadvantage is that computer activities can easily become a dominant obsession; from the start, parents should impose clear limits on the time allowed in these activities.

It is worth trying to engage autistic children in simple games. Singing games with actions are likely to be enjoyed. Most children enjoy chasing games though they have difficulty in understanding the concept of taking turns to chase and be chased. They may be able to learn to play hide-and-seek when they have sufficient understanding to know that objects still exist if they are hidden away. It is best to begin by playing with one of the child's favorite possessions. One helper can cover the child's eyes or take them out of the room while the other helper does the hiding. The child will need to be helped to search and the object will have to be "found" quickly at first in order to avoid causing upset through failure. As the child begins to see the point and to enjoy the surprise element, the game can go on longer and they can be encouraged to search for themselves. The child will tend to go back to the same place over and over again and will need cues to other possible hiding places. Most of the very simple games enjoyed by young children can be adapted to include a child with an autistic disorder. The experience is particularly valuable if other children can join in but they usually need adult guidance to help them adapt to the level of the child with the autistic disorder.

Some of the children reach the level at which they can play picture-matching games or board games such as Snakes and Ladders. Some of the most able learn to play chess and do well because of their excellent visuo-spatial memories. When young, most of the children have no concept of winning or losing and board games give the opportunity to teach this. The trouble is, if and when they do learn, they may become very upset or angry and have a major temper tantrum if they lose. Board games at home with the family can be useful in teaching a show of good grace when losing, if the nerves of everyone concerned can stand living through the learning process.

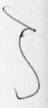

The hardest problem is to keep up the children's interest in any activity. Other children are eager to try out their developing understanding of the social and physical world. Children with autistic disorders lack this drive because they have no comprehension of what life is about. They need supervision and encouragement to prevent them from filling all their time with repetitive routines.

Physical Activities

Since children with autistic disorders have little capacity for creative play, it is especially useful to encourage physical activities that are enjoyable without the need for imagination and use of language. Physical exercise is also reported to diminish inappropriate behavior. Such activities are also helpful for improving the problems of motor coordination so often seen in autistic disorders.

The children usually enjoy listening and moving to music, walking and running, sand and water play, swings, merry-go-rounds, slides and climbing structures. Many learn to swim even though they cannot take part in any other sport. Horseback riding, supervised by qualified instructors who are experienced in working with disabled people, often proves to be a special pleasure. If there is access to sessions in a gymnasium, autistic children may enjoy using some of the apparatus, especially trampolines, and may achieve surprising levels of skill. Here too, qualified instructors must be present to supervise. Many children eventually learn to ride tricycles or bicycles, with or without stabilizers. Most are happy when riding in cars or other forms of transportation. Even adventurous pursuits such as rock-climbing may be attempted providing they are organized and supervised by instructors who are trained, experienced and understand the needs of people with autistic disorders. Some of the more-able learn to play games that involve only two people, such as table tennis.

Difficulties may arise in playgrounds open to all children. Those with autistic disorders may run straight into swings being used by other children without being aware of the danger. They may have no idea about taking turns and push other children out of the way or even off the equipment. When this behavior is stopped, there may be temper tantrums and screaming. It is important for those supervising to be calm and adamant that difficult or dangerous behavior will be prevented, if necessary by removing the child from the playground as soon as problems arise.

Poor motor coordination tends to reduce the children's opportunities for physical exercise. Some skills can be taught by helping the child to physically move hands, arms and legs appropriately. The guidance can be reduced bit by bit until it is no longer needed. Riding a tricycle, for example, can be taught in this way. Another problem can be fear that inhibits a child from trying some activities. The gradual desensitization approach as described in Chapter 9 can be used to overcome the anxiety.

Children with Profound Learning Difficulties

Among the range of children with autistic disorders, there are some who have very severe or profound learning difficulties and whose capacity for progress is very limited. Their disabilities are shown by their lack of practical skills in everyday life and their poor performance on psychological testing. As with all children with autistic disorders, their real level of ability becomes clearer with increasing age and no firm decision should be made before five years old at the earliest. There are occasional children who have one or two specific visuo-spatial skills, such as dexterity with jigsaw puzzles or who can chatter repetitively, but have no other skills at all. These children can be a puzzle because they appear to have more ability than is in fact the case. If psychological testing reveals that they have profound learning difficulties, they also will need the type of program to be described below.

Applying pressure to make any of these children perform tasks above their level of ability produces no useful result and may lead to temper tantrums, negativism, aggression towards others, or self-injury. An organized daily program of activities in which they can participate is essential to help them enjoy a reasonable quality of life and to make life easier for the whole family.

The important skills for them to acquire, as much as they possibly can, are those of basic self-care, especially toilet training and self-feeding. These should be taught in very small steps, with gentle physical prompting, as a regular part of each day.

The types of leisure pursuits they can enjoy are the physical activities described above. Despite the children's very severe disabilities, some of them achieve surprising levels of skill in one or more of these activities, given patience and gentle persistence from the instructor.

The development of "Snoezelen" rooms, with equipment that provides stimulation to the senses of sight, hearing, smell, touch, as well as vibration and movement has been of benefit to children with severe impairments, including those with autistic disorders. The same kinds of activities, suitably modified for a mature age and larger size, are appropriate for adults with profound learning difficulties.

Physical Health

Autistic children should be taught as best as they are able basic rules of hygiene, including teeth cleaning and care. Those who are less able will need to be supervised in all health matters and the most disabled will need complete care.

As described in Chapter 11, those children who have problems with chewing or who insist on a diet limited to sweet foods can be susceptible to gum disease and tooth decay. Careful and regular tooth brushing is essential. If the child will accept it, an electric toothbrush, if used properly, cleans effectively and also helps the child to become used to the feeling of vibration in the mouth, which is similar to that of some dental instruments. Regular visits to the dentist are necessary and should begin well before any treatment is needed.

Writers on health matters usually stress the importance of a balanced and varied diet. This rule can be difficult to apply to the many children with autistic disorders who eat only what they decide they will and generally show no symptoms of dietary deficiency, doubtless to the chagrin of the diet fanatics.

As already mentioned, physical exercise is helpful in many ways for children with autistic disorders, especially from the point of view of physical fitness.

Most of the children are active and energetic and have few illnesses. There are some who have various conditions due to allergies, including asthma. It has been suggested that allergies are a cause of autism but no firm evidence for this has been published. If the autistic disorder is associated with a physical disorder, such as tuberose sclerosis, appropriate treatment and supervision will be needed for this.

Epileptic seizures occur in a substantial minority of people with autistic disorders. If they do, investigations are needed to search for any underlying physical cause. Medication need not be started immediately. If the seizures happen only with a fever, or if only one or two occur and no underlying cause or EEG abnormality is found, then medication may not be needed. However, if medication to control recurrent seizures is needed, there should be regular monitoring of its effectiveness and possible side effects.

The problems of communication, especially expressing feelings, make it difficult for children with autistic disorders to indicate when they do not feel well, or to show the site of any pain. As described earlier, they can appear not to notice even severe pain. Parents often have to deduce that the child is unwell by observation of such behavior as extra fretfulness, lack of appetite, lethargy, rashes or a feverish flush. This can occur even in more-able children with good language. If the child has some speech, it is useful to teach a few words that can be used if they are in pain or discomfort. "Throat sore" or "Leg hurt," does give some guide to what is wrong. A small girl liked to have a Band-aid put on any minor injury. When she had an attack of tonsillitis the first sign was when she said to her mother, "Poor froat—put Band-aid on."

Many young autistic children furiously resist attempts at physical examination although some may happily accept medical procedures when they are older. Practicing a physical examination as part of a game with parents or siblings at home sometimes can help the child accept it more easily. This can include making the child accustomed to the feeling of a cold stethoscope on the chest, using a similar-sized metal object such as the end of a flashlight. It is also useful to practice opening and closing the eyes and the mouth when told. If possible, the child should get to know the family doctor as a friend before any treatment is needed so that there is less apprehension when the child does become ill. Unfortunately, the busy schedule of most family doctors makes this difficult.

If a child has to go into the hospital it is usually better if a parent or other caretaker can accompany them. The child with an autistic disorder is likely to be very disturbed by being in a strange place and needs the reassurance of the presence of a familiar person. Any toys or objects that the child clings to should be brought as well. The doctors and nurses will need the parent's help to explain and give instructions in a way the child understands. The parent can also tell the staff of the child's needs since the children often cannot convey their meaning to strangers. The doctor and charge nurse may appreciate some information about children with autistic conditions if they have not treated a child with this disability before. In this situation parents have to hide their natural anxiety, present a calm and confident front to their child and cooperate fully with the medical and nursing staff so that the child feels as happy and relaxed as possible. Despite their social and communication impairments, many children with autistic conditions are remarkably good at picking up small signs of unhappy emotions in other people.

A doctor or dentist who is treating a child should be told if the child is receiving any medication of any kind. This is particularly important if an anesthetic, local or general, has to be given. Children with autistic conditions may be muddled and confused when they wake up from an anesthetic. They will be helped and comforted if a parent or another familiar person is there to give reassurance. Some children with autistic conditions are unusually resistant to sedatives, pre-medication or anesthetics. In some cases these excite rather than sedate them. This possibility should be mentioned to medical or dental staff who are treating the child.

The uses and problems of medication were mentioned in Chapter 11. If medication is prescribed, parents should ask for detailed information about the reasons for prescribing the medication, the dosage and method of administration, when it should begin to act, possible side effects, how to detect them and what to do if they occur. Be sure to find out if there are special things to avoid, such as sunlight or particular foods, and how long the medication will be continued.

CHAPTER 13

Babies with Autistic Spectrum Disorders

Autistic disorders are usually not diagnosed until the age of two or later, so no one can recommend well-tried methods of dealing with the problems in babies. If ever a reliable method of making a diagnosis in infancy is developed, it will then be possible to test ideas in practice. This chapter is included in case there are readers who suspect that a baby they know may have an autistic disorder, perhaps because of the behavior pattern and a family history.

The interactions of babies with their parents should be a two-way process, with the baby contributing eagerness for and pleasure in response to the attention. This rewards the parents and helps to strengthen the mutual bonds. Babies who have autistic behavior from birth tend not to show enjoyment of or even the need for social attention so parents are not rewarded in the usual way for their efforts. It says much for the strength of parental feelings in human beings that most keep trying. It seems reasonable to suggest that if a baby is undemanding or rejecting of some forms of contact, the parents should observe the things that do seem to give pleasure and use these when caring or playing. Most such babies like active physical play such as tickling or bouncing up and down. They also usually love music, so singing or playing favorite tapes while dressing, washing, or changing can help the baby accept these procedures with less protest.

Many children with autistic disorders pay more attention to words that are sung to a tune than those that are spoken. The same seems likely to be true of the babies. Some show enjoyment if words are whispered into their ears—it may be the tickling sensation they like but, whatever the reason, it is a good idea to associate words with pleasurable feelings.

Parents often remember that fascination with particular stimuli, such as lights, television, a special sound or object, started during the first year of life. Some recall that the babies could be absorbed in these experiences for long periods of time. No one knows the long-term effect of either allowing this or preventing it. Again, it seems a sensible idea to compromise by allowing enjoyment of these activities for a time but then to intervene to try to involve the baby in more sociable play. The same goes for a baby who is content to be alone much of the time. The aim should be to make social interactions positively rewarding for the baby in whatever way can be found, but to stop before boredom or resistance begins.

From parents' accounts, it appears that most babies who are later recognized to have an autistic disorder are quiet and undemanding. Babies who scream much of the time are in a minority. The hardest thing for parents of babies like this is that cuddling does not soothe and may even make things worse. Most discover that walking around, rocking and singing to the baby are helpful, as are the movements of a stroller or a car. The problem is that the screaming starts again as soon as the movement stops and may go on through the night. There is no fund of advice that is guaranteed to be of help with such babies. Parents, especially if it is their first child, are often made to feel inadequate by others who criticize them because they "cannot manage the baby." The critics would experience an equal lack of success if they tried to care for the child.

If the baby does not sleep and cries a great deal at night, sometimes music or a low continuous mechanical sound may prove helpful. Leaving a light on or, conversely, excluding light may induce the baby to settle down. But none of these remedies is guaranteed to work. The degree of exhaustion experienced by the parents can be reduced if it is possible for them to take turns or to involve someone else who is able to take a share of night care.

As with all other age groups, a regular, predictable routine for each day is the aim. This is relatively easy to achieve with the quiet babies but much more difficult with those who cry or scream a great deal and who are awake at night.

CHAPTER 14

Adolescents and Adults Who Remain Dependent

Variations in the pattern of skills and behavior are even wider among adolescents and adults than among children with autistic disorders. At one end of the spectrum, some change so little that they still have the same problems as those of the young child. At the other end are adolescents who have progressed so much that they are in mainstream education and are likely to become independent as adults. For these children, the problems faced in adolescence have something in common with those of other teenagers in addition to the special difficulties arising from the autistic impairments.

The special needs of those who are more able will be discussed in a later section. Here, the focus will be on those who remain dependent all their lives.

Adolescents

Inappropriate Behavior

Many, though not all, of the more disabled adolescents show an exacerbation of difficult behavior in the teenage years. The physiological changes that lead to puberty and increase in physical size also produce psychological changes. It seems that, even in those who are most severely disabled and unaware of social situations, adolescence brings a reluctance to accept adult authority and a determination not to give in. In those with limited ability, these feelings may be shown in a return to temper tantrums, aggression and other behaviors of the early years. It is much harder for parents to cope with a tantrum in someone who is bigger and stronger than they are and is aware of the fact. Immature behavior in a teenager also attracts more adverse reactions in public than the same behavior in a small child.

Head-on confrontations are even less likely to produce useful results with an adolescent than they are with a child. Both at home and at school, careful planning is required. Just as in childhood, the program for each day should be organized, predictable and presented in visual form. Within this framework, the activities and demands made on a teenager have to be adjusted to take into account the changes in age, interests and attitudes. It may be best, if it is possible, to avoid situations where problems are likely to occur.

Education

The educational program should be planned to help develop skills that will be useful in adult life. Special schools are generally privately run. Age criteria varies a great deal depending on the school. Some may offer services only until middle school (age 12), while many allow children to stay through age 21.

Cooperation between home and school in organizing activities and responding consistently to inappropriate behavior is of great value. It may be that the behavior is very different in the two environments. Usually, if there is a difference, the behavior is calmer and more cooperative at school than at home, but it can be the other way around. There is a temptation to blame those in charge where the difficulties occur but this is unjustifiable and not constructive. An exchange of ideas and mutual support is much more helpful.

Leisure Activities

Inappropriate behavior is always less likely when the individual is occupied. Teenagers with autistic disorders, like all young adults, tend to lose interest in the childish activities they enjoyed when younger. The problem is that those who are less able have no interest in the activities that fill the lives of other adults and they cannot find constructive occupations for themselves. Parents and teachers have to explore all the possibilities for occupation and leisure that may be interesting and enjoyable to the individual concerned. Physical activities of all kinds are among the most likely to appeal. Computers may still hold their fascination and art work, pottery, weaving, gardening, domestic work and other practical occupations have been enjoyed by some teens. The aim is to develop an atmosphere of cooperation and give and take that is appropriate for those who are becoming adults. At the same time, parents and teachers have to retain sufficient control to maintain the all-important structure for each day and to keep the teenager with an autistic disorder safe and in good health. Keeping the right balance is not an easy task.

Sexual Development

Puberty is usually not delayed in children with autistic disorders even though they often look younger than their actual age. Interest in the social aspects of sexual relationships requires more language and social understanding than most teenagers with autistic disorders, who will remain dependent all their lives, have acquired. Some develop a curiosity about other people's bodies and may try to touch and look in inappropriate ways or even try to undress other children. This should be stopped immediately but without any display of negative emotion. Most, sooner or later, discover how to masturbate. The rule must be that this is done only in private. Again, it is essential to react calmly, conveying the rule with clarity but without anger or distress. There has been some discussion among parents and professionals as to the desirability of teaching someone with an autistic disorder to masturbate to orgasm if they are showing signs of sexual arousal and do not seem to know how to obtain relief. The problems associated with this, and the emotional complications of embarking on such a program, are too great for this to be advisable.

Menstruation usually begins within the same age range as with other girls. Most girls seem to accept this without much concern. Perhaps to a girl with an autistic disorder, it is just one more inexplicable event in a puzzling world. A routine for changing pads regularly should be followed with the aim of teaching the girl eventually to care for herself. Sometimes a teenager will talk about her periods to people she meets. Although it is an excellent idea to adopt an open and matter-of-fact attitude towards the facts of life, it is necessary to teach discretion in these matters because there are still many people who are shocked or embarrassed by these subjects. You can explain that the time to make comments or ask questions is when they are alone with their parents or other caregivers and not when other people are around. As always, the calm approach is essential.

Asking questions about conception and birth presupposes a reasonable level of language development, so it is only a small minority of the more dependent adolescents who will even ask their parents about these matters. Answers should be frank, but simple enough for the teenager's understanding. Rules for socially acceptable behavior in these matters should be included in the discussion.

Some adolescents with autistic disorders are naively friendly to everyone and are easily led. Some girls are particularly likely to approach men and may show physical affection indiscriminately. Parents and other caregivers are properly concerned about the dangers that could ensue. Most girls with autistic disorders who remain highly dependent can be supervised closely enough to avoid problems of sexual encounters. However, if there is the possibility of an undesirable contact occurring, the question of prescribing a contraceptive pill or other contraceptive measure has to be considered. It must also be kept in mind that some teenage boys with autistic disorders could be vulnerable to sexual abuse.

Adults

People with autistic disorders tend to look and behave much younger than their years. The concerns of adolescence continue long into adult life. Eventually, increasing age tends to bring calmer and more appropriate behavior after the turmoil of adolescence, though it is not possible to say for any individual when this is likely to occur.

Occupation

After school, it is essential for adults with autistic disorders to have a regular, daily occupation. A few of those who are dependent on others are able to work at simple, routine jobs in paid employment. The great majority require sheltered work in day centers. As with all other aspects of life, the work available needs to be suitable for the abilities and interests and attention span of the individual. The daily timetable needs to be structured and clearly set out in visual terms with adequate help and supervision available from trained staff. The work environment should be calm, quiet and should provide enough personal space. This is particularly important for many people with autistic disorders. Of course, these are the ideal conditions. The types of centers that actually exist and the problems of obtaining a place need to be explored.

Leaving Home

A small minority of children and adolescents with autistic disorders attend boarding school for the latter part of their school life. However, most go to day schools and live at home during school-age years. Parents have to give careful thought to the question of where their children will live when they become adults. It is necessary to start thinking some years before the child becomes 18 years old because good residential places are in short supply.

Many parents find it difficult to think about the possibility of their children leaving home and being cared for by strangers. They know they understand their child better than anyone else and they worry endlessly about what will happen when their son or daughter no longer has the protection of home and family. Despite the emotional distress, parents need to face the fact that they will not always be able to care for their child. Their circumstances may change for any number of reasons, making it essential to find residential care for the person with an autistic disorder. The needs of sisters and brothers who are living at home, as well as the quality of life of the parents themselves, have to be considered. It is much better to plan in advance and, if possible, to see the child settled into a home while the parents still have their health and strength to find the best placement so they can take action if a particular home is chosen and then found unsuitable. Furthermore, the transition is eased if the parents can have their son or daughter home for weekends, frequently at first, and then less often as they settle in.

From the point of view of the young adult with an autistic disorder there are advantages in leaving home. This, after all, is the most usual pattern of life. They will meet different people, have access to new experiences, some of which they will enjoy. They may learn new skills and more adaptive behavior and be able to take part in a wider range of leisure activities. Often, but by no means always, there is a difficult period of settling in, which lasts for varying lengths of time. If the environment is right, this passes and life becomes easier and more enjoyable.

CHAPTER 15

The More-Able Children,
Adolescents and Adults

Definition and Diagnosis

I am including in this group the children, adolescents and adults who have language and non-verbal skills ranging from low-average to superior. The epidemiological study that was carried out in Sweden, as mentioned in Chapter 4, suggests that around 7 in every 1000 children in the general population have this type of developmental disorder.

Some of those who are more able during infancy and early childhood show the behavior pattern of typical autism. As they grow older, language and other skills develop well and they become more and more like the Asperger group. Others fit Asperger's syndrome from the beginning, having no delay in language or adaptive skills. Whatever their early history, by the time of adolescence or early adulthood most have most or all of the features described by Asperger —repetitive speech and active but naive social interaction. A small minority retain more of the characteristics of Kanner's syndrome, being socially aloof and uncommunicative despite good comprehension and use of language on psychological testing. Yet others fit neither of these syndromes but have a mix of features clearly within the autistic spectrum.

As explained in Chapter 2, the latest versions of the international classifications ICD-10 and DSM-IV have as an essential criterion for Asperger's syndrome the absence of delay in development of language and other adaptive skills. In clinical practice, as distinct from research, it is the person's current pattern of behavior that determines the needs rather than their early history. It is more important to recognize that someone has an autistic spectrum disorder and to assess their level and pattern of ability than to argue about which sub-group they belong to.

Childhood

The children who have typical autistic behavior in their early years are likely to be recognized as having a developmental disorder even if the correct diagnosis is not made. The problems and needs of those who begin to talk at the usual age and whose self-care and practical skills develop more-or-less normally are often unrecognized until major problems occur at school. Many are not diagnosed until adolescence or adulthood, if ever.

Early recognition of the nature of the children's disabilities is as necessary for those who are more able as it is for those with more severe disabilities. The more-able children are impaired in their understanding of the nature of social interaction, are unable to use their good speech for true reciprocal communication and are rigid and repetitive in their imagination and pattern of activities. They have the same basic impairments as the more severely affected children but manifest them in somewhat different ways. They also have the same need for a structured, organized program and for a timetable to provide a framework for each day.

Problems at Home and at School

There are some more-able children who have a gentle, amenable temperament. Most, however, have an intense determination to do what they want to do regardless of any considerations. They are unconcerned about the consequences of their actions, whether they affect other people or themselves. This is probably due to an inability to foresee consequences, to weigh the pros and cons and to make sensible plans for the future. The absence of these skills is probably a direct consequence of the neuropathology that underlies autistic spectrum disorders.

That same singlemindedness often leads to difficulties at school. If a correct diagnosis has not been made, the child's stubborn refusal to do anything that does not interest them and their habit of saying exactly what they think can easily be interpreted as cheeky disobedience. They tend to be unpopular with other children because they do not share the interests of their age peers and are recognized as odd and different. The undiagnosed bright child with an autistic disorder can be intensely unhappy at school. Some do not know how to tell anyone of their misery and endure in silence. Some are aggressive with their peers, who often torment them, and are then in further trouble. Some refuse to go to school and some, in adolescence, have a depressive reaction or other psychiatric illness.

Another characteristic that can cause difficulties at home and at school is the tendency to talk on and on about the same subject, or to ask repetitive questions regardless of the answers or, most irritating of all, to engage in arguments that are endless because the child always finds a new objection to whatever is suggested.

Making Life Easier

Living with someone with an autistic disorder who has good language and skills is, on balance, more difficult than living with someone who is more severely disabled and obviously dependent on others. The more-able older children and adolescents often want to be as independent as their age peers and are unwilling to accept parental authority. Some suggestions can be made to smooth the path a little for parents and teachers.

At Home

Most of the points made in this section are applicable at school as well as at home.

It is important to make the essential home or school rules very clear and to make sure the child understands that they are applicable to everyone. The children are resentful if they think they are being unfairly picked on, but are more likely to follow rules that are to be obeyed by everyone in the family or the class. Asperger wrote that his children were more willing to obey rules that were expressed as universally applicable rather than directed at them specifically. "Everyone in this house, (school, family) must. . . ." The drawback is that once stated in this way the child with the autistic disorder will be the first to notice and object if someone else breaks the rule. They are less concerned about their own violations.

Never become angry or emotional. This is easy to say, difficult to do, but very helpful if you can. Remain cool, detached, judicious and absolutely fair to all. Autistic children cannot cope with strong emotions, whether in themselves or other people. Faced with overt emotion, they tend to become distressed, angry and negative in re-action. Particularly distressing to parents is the fact that the more-able children do not respond to appeals to act or behave in particular ways in order to please or to spare their parents' feelings. The children cannot empathize because they have little or no capacity to understand other people's thoughts and feelings. Many parents have been deeply hurt by the apparent lack of feeling in their child. This is yet another reason why an early diagnosis is so important. When parents are given a full explanation of the nature of autistic disorders, they find it much easier to accept their child's apparent callousness. They can then begin to develop a more objective, non-emotional approach that works much better.

Avoid head-on confrontation whenever possible. The children will always win an open battle because they have no built-in submission to authority or desire to please. Furthermore, punishment will not deter them. Negotiation and compromise are more helpful. If it is absolutely essential that they obey an edict, then the adult in charge has to be calmly implacable and indifferent to the child's techniques of opposition. Endless patience is required because it can take a very long time.

Avoid involvement in arguments. Some children are skilled at finding loopholes in every point you make and you cannot win. The same is true if they want to pursue questions on a particular topic. One way to terminate a discussion that is getting nowhere is to say, calmly but firmly, that the subject is now closed. Sometimes it is helpful to give a child a precise amount of time, perhaps five minutes, in which to ask questions or discuss a situation. You must stick rigidly to this.

Most children with autistic conditions, especially those who are more able, continually test the boundaries laid down by parents and teachers. Some appear to deliberately tease and defy. However, this trait is not due to "naughtiness" but occurs from the lack of development of an internalized system of rules for social interaction. The testing behavior is minimized in environments that are structured and organized, where the rules are fair and given in ways that are absolutely clear to the children and where the adult authority figures are calm and consistent in their approach and follow the same line. The aim is to help the children develop over time some internalized rules for living, even though these tend to be rigid and inflexible.

The children do not understand ambiguity or double meanings and take everything literally. They are confused by sarcasm or irony, which should be avoided when talking to them.

The needs of brothers and sisters are important but can be overlooked by parents struggling to cope with a child with an autistic disorder. This subject is discussed in more detail in Chapter 16.

AT SCHOOL

The points made below are particularly relevant for children attending mainstream schools or other types of school that do not specialize in teaching children with autistic disorders. The advantages and disadvantages of different types of schooling are discussed in Chapter 16.

The children have no concept of hierarchy based on age, class, lines of authority or anything else—they are natural democrats. They say what they think with no regard for other people's feelings, or for the consequences. These attributes, which have their admirable side, even if infuriating at times, are not due to rebelliousness or cheekiness. It helps to be aware of this and to avoid getting annoyed.

Despite their apparent self-assurance and indifference to authority, most more-able children with autistic disorders have a very low self-esteem even if they are of high ability. They have all experienced many failures in social interaction and are sensitive to the laughter and scorn of their age peers when they behave in a naive way. Some develop a paranoid attitude as a result. These sensitivities should be kept in mind when teaching or caring for the children.

It helps to take every opportunity to involve the more-able children in pursuits that raise their self-esteem, such as physical activities they are good at (if any), music, or taking part in quizzes that need a good rote memory. Some (though not all) of the children have no fear and love performing in front of an audience. Finding them the right type of part in a school play or other special occasion and giving them enough coaching can be most rewarding for all concerned.

Most of the children like to be praised. However, there are a few who, paradoxically, become angry and negative if praised for anything, even though they have poor self-esteem. There is no known explanation for this, unless it is a dislike of being picked out as different. If a child has this trait, care has to be taken to avoid verbal commendation. Non-verbal ways of showing approval should be tried.

The children often do not realize that when the whole group is addressed they are included. It is necessary to ensure that their attention is gained in class. When doing this, it is important to remember their sensitivity to being picked out unfairly, so gaining their attention has to be done tactfully.

It is important to find ways to use the children's positive skills in learning and not to concentrate on the things they cannot do. The desire to learn can often be encouraged by working with the child's special interests and linking teaching with these interests as much as possible. For example, with some ingenuity, a fascination with trains could be utilized in teaching art, physics, mathematics, English, geography, even history. If, however, there is a particular subject that a child refuses even to try to learn, it is best to compromise. The child can be allowed to pursue a personal interest quietly for that particular time as long as the rest of the class is not disturbed.

Various kinds of specific learning disorders are often associated with autistic conditions in more-able children. These should be identified by psychological assessment so that they can be addressed in the teaching plan. Some of the children are much better at visuo-spatial skills than at understanding language, even if they have fluent speech. For such children, presenting concepts in visual form rather than verbal terms is very helpful. Some, on the other hand, have specific visuo-spatial difficulties but have better expressive language, though they usually have problems with aspects of language comprehension. Teaching has to be adjusted to help them cope with these problems.

Poor physical coordination is common, though by no means universal. This may be present for most motor activities, even though the child has some special skill that does require good coordination, such as playing a musical instrument or making constructional toys. For those with poor coordination in large movements, team games can be a nightmare. Efforts should be made to find some kind of physical activity that is within the child's capacity so that they can hold their own with their age peers in at least one pursuit.

Break times and lunch hours in school are particularly stressful for autistic children because they are unstructured. Supervision is necessary to ensure that they do not become distressed, or engage in bizarre, stereotyped behavior. They may cope better if allowed to stay inside working on a computer or doing something else that they like. If they are outside with the other children they need to be protected from bullying and teasing. It may be necessary to explain to other children something about the problem and to call on their sympathy. The way to do this is to emphasize the child's special gifts as well as their problems. This should always be done, if at all, in consultation and with the agreement of the parents and, if appropriate, the child concerned.

Not all of the children have a bad time in mainstream schools or schools for a mix of disabilities. Some of the children have a special skill that may be admired by their classmates, such as playing a musical instrument, math abilities, or dexterity with constructional kits. Some who are quiet and gentle are befriended by another child and thereby enjoy a protector. It requires good supervision and observation to discover how the children with autistic disorders are coping because of their inability to express their own feelings.

Adolescence

As with all children with autistic disorders, adolescence may bring a period of disturbed behavior in some, though in others it can be the time when progress is accelerated. The problems that occur tend to be related to four particular concerns: desire for independence; increasing awareness of their disability; wanting friendships and sexual relationships; and pressures of exams at school.

Desire for Independence

Regardless of the level of ability, adolescence is associated with increasing size, strength and assertiveness. Those who are more able often want the same freedoms as their age peers, even though they are naive, immature and are not at all street-wise. Ideally, home and school should cooperate in teaching rules for sensible conduct so that some freedom can be allowed. This teaching has to begin early and be carried on for years. It helps, but no list of rules can ever be long enough to cover all possible situations that are met in real life. With the more-able group, parents have to accept some risks because they cannot keep a determined teenager under their supervision all the time. All they can do is to make the rules of conduct outside the home as clear as possible and to teach the young person where to turn for help in an emergency.

The more-able adolescents with autistic disorders, especially those with Asperger syndrome, sometimes show their growing assertiveness by blaming their parents for all their troubles, despite all the love and care they have received throughout their childhood. They may give trivial or bizarre reasons for their hostility towards their parents. One teenager, for example, said that all his difficulties were due to the fact that his parents would not buy him an extremely expensive computer that he wanted when he was eight years old.

Such accusations can make parents feel guilty even if they know they are irrational. The best way for parents to cope is to remain calm and to refuse to be drawn into arguments and justifications of their actions. If the hostility becomes intense and cannot be resolved, it may be best to seek some form of accommodation away from home, such as a residential school (see Chapter 16).

A small minority of more-able adolescents are so determined to have their own way that they try to dominate others in the family. In a few cases, the individual is so domineering that others in the family have no life of their own. They have to fit in with the often bizarre, repetitive pattern of life imposed on them in order to avoid temper tantrums and aggressive behavior. In all cases of this kind that I have met, the diagnosis of an autistic disorder, usually Asperger's syndrome, has not been made in childhood so the family is bewildered by the behavior of the individual concerned. When the diagnosis is made in early childhood, it is possible for the parents and teachers to provide the necessary structured and organized environment and to lay down and enforce sensible rules before adolescence begins.

Once this type of situation has developed, the only recourse for the parents is to ask for help from social services and psychiatric services through referral by the family doctor. Sorting out the diagnosis is the first priority, before any action to relieve the stress on the family can be initiated. It is important for parents to tell the whole story to professionals involved. They should not try to hide the full extent of the difficulties in an effort to protect their disabled son or daughter, who is just as damaged by being allowed to dominate the home as are the rest of the family. In most cases, the only solution is some form of residential provision away from home (see Chapter 16).

In his first paper, Asperger noted that individuals with his syndrome tend to be strongly attached to their own homes. The attachment is to the physical surroundings rather than to the family. This sometimes leads to intense dislike of leaving home, even for an overnight stay, and even more so for a longer vacation. It is paradoxical that a desire for personal independence can be combined with a refusal to leave the family home. When it is present in marked form, the attachment to home can make vacations a misery for the whole family. With teenagers or adults who can manage on their own for a few days, it may be best to leave them at home while the rest of the family takes a break. This problem does not occur in everyone with Asperger's syndrome. Some love journeys and new places and are at their best on vacations when there is plenty to occupy them.

Awareness of Disability

It is difficult to know how aware young children are of their disabilities. They certainly feel intense distress when they are frustrated or confused by their environment. The more-able children are likely to have a fair amount of insight by the time they reach adolescence. They may express this in their own way. One boy used to say, very sadly, when he failed at some task, "Can't do it. Got no brain." A girl of 14 once asked her mother, "Mommy, when God made me why didn't he make me quite right?" Some teenagers want to know why they are different from their siblings or their age peers. The response to developing insight varies, depending upon the personality and temperament of each individual. Some accept without becoming distressed, some become unhappy and depressed and some try to cope by denying that they have any problems and becoming angry if the subject is mentioned.

The young people who accept without concern are the most fortunate and easiest to live with. Those who react with distress need support from their family and others with whom they have close contact. Occasionally adolescents with autistic disorders who are concerned about themselves will do something inappropriate to overcome their problems. One young man suddenly decided he could improve his health if he took up running, so he promptly set out and ran for miles in bitterly cold weather in his undershirt and underwear and was found in an exhausted condition a long way from home. It may not be possible to predict, and therefore prevent, this kind of impulsive behavior. It is also impossible to shield more-able adolescents from the knowledge that they do have problems that are not shared by most other people.

In order to improve their self-esteem, their positive skills should be emphasized and praised. It is often helpful to point out, as Asperger did, that there are many other people who are like them and some are high achievers in art or science. Some ask if they have a "mental illness." It is reasonable to explain that the basic problem is not an illness but a different type of organization of the brain that has advantages as well as disadvantages. It can be pointed out that everyone is good at some things and less good at others. The more-able person with autism is poor at understanding other people and expressing their own feelings, but is good in some other areas. It may help them to know that many people admire and envy the special skills that the person with an autistic disorder does have. An explanation of this kind can be tailored to suit each individual, taking into account their level of understanding. In the course of everyday life, their help should be elicited in situations in which their special skills can be put to good use.

It is difficult to help the adolescents who deny their disability even though it is obvious that beneath the surface they are aware and unhappy. Any attempt at a discussion along the lines suggested above tends to provoke rage and further denial. The only course of action is to say nothing but to be prepared to give support if and when the individual shows the need.

Friendships and Sexual Relationships

Some more-able adolescents are unconcerned that they have no friends and are not interested in having a girl or boy friend. Others realize that they have great difficulty in forming relationships and cope by deciding that they are not going to try. The majority are very aware of and distressed by their inability to form friendships, or to maintain them if they are ever started. Their capacity to comprehend the meaning and nature of friendship is often limited. They lack the instinctive knowledge of how to make the first moves prior to becoming accepted by others. If they do begin a relationship, they are often unable to give and take and may make inappropriate demands on the other person.

As in all other spheres of life, the adolescent with an autistic disorder has to be taught the basic rules of social interaction with age peers, which are not easy to formulate. Joining clubs or groups can be a source of pleasure and helps in developing social skills. This is likely to work best if the group caters to the interests of the individual concerned. Locomotive clubs may attract those who are fascinated by trains. Chess clubs are excellent for the enthusiasts of this game. Social clubs that are not dedicated to a particular pursuit are less likely to be acceptable. Sometimes friendships do develop between group members with similar personalities and interests. In such cases, they tend to talk at each other about their particular subject, happily reeling off lists of train numbers or details of chess games without any true conversational exchange.

On the whole, the desire for a girl or boy friend is motivated more by the wish to copy what most other people of their age do rather than the need for an emotional relationship. Nevertheless, there is often a strong determination to succeed. Many of the young people have asked parents or teachers if there are books that will tell them how to get a partner and how to talk to them. To increase the difficulties, the boys often have very specific requirements for a girlfriend, such as long blonde hair and blue eyes. The girls do not seem to be as choosy.

Establishing this sort of relationship is far harder than starting an ordinary friendship. If a teenage boy does find a girlfriend, she often terminates the relationship in a short time because she soon realizes how odd he is, or how socially gauche, and how little he is aware of her emotional or practical needs. For example, a 17-year-old boy with an autistic disorder made friends with a younger girl, whom he regarded as his special girlfriend. His mother suggested that it would please the girl if he gave her a birthday present. "All right," said the boy, "I will if she gives me the money." He was very surprised when she ceased to have anything to do with him. Apart from teaching social skills as far as is possible, providing emotional support and pointing out that many people live satisfying lives without a sexual partner, little can be done to help.

If there is a specific interest in the physical aspects of sex, teaching rules concerning appropriate behavior is particularly important. As much supervision as possible with regard to the individual's age and level of ability should also be organized. Indiscriminate displays of affection or naive encouragement of physical contact, such as touching and tickling, should be firmly discouraged when they are inappropriate. If for any reason a girl is particularly vulnerable and cannot be supervised all the time, advice on contraception should be sought.

Pressure of Exams

Some adolescents have no problems and do well academically. Others find the work at high school level increasingly difficult. They kept up with the rest of the class, ostensibly at least, at the primary stage because they used their good rote memories. Secondary education requires adequate understanding of what is learned and the ability to make connections and draw conclusions rather than just remembering. When preparations for exams begin, some of the pupils with autistic disorders experience high levels of stress. This causes some to give up and refuse to attend school. One teenager took to his bed and would not get up. Some struggle on without complaint but do poorly in the exams. Others develop behavior problems or a diagnosable psychiatric illness, usually depression (see below, under "Adult Life"), before or during the exams. Very few return to school after such an event.

Early diagnosis, accurate assessment of the child's level of ability and placement in the most appropriate type of school help to avoid later problems due to exam pressures. When exams approach, sensitive supervision and careful observation by teachers and parents help to detect early signs of trouble. Special facilities for taking exams, perhaps with a known supervisor and away from the large examination hall, may be sufficient. Modifications such as untimed testing can sometimes be arranged for individuals taking standardized tests such as the Scholastic Aptitude Test (SAT). However, un-timed tests are flagged as such when scores are reported to colleges. This may or may not have an impact on how the scores are inter-preted by an admissions committee.

If the problems are too severe to solve in such ways, it is best to allow the young person to drop out altogether rather than risk a severe breakdown. If a breakdown of the kind to be described below does occur, then the exams cannot be taken.

Adult Life

The major concerns for more-able adults with autistic disorders are living accommodation, employment and whether or not they can marry or live with a partner and start a family.

Living Accommodations

Considering the whole range of autistic disorders, including those with high levels of skill and no disabilities except for the triad of impairments in the most subtle form, it is possible to say with some confidence that the majority of the most-able adults are capable of living independently. That still leaves a large number who do not develop sufficient self-care, domestic and practical skills, or com-mon sense, to have their own homes.

A proportion continue to live with their parents. This may work fairly well if the individual concerned has regular sheltered or open employment, some leisure activities and is reasonably helpful and cooperative in the home. Some, however, have no outside activities of any kind because they have no paid work and there is no employ-ment that is suitable in their local area. In such cases, the adult stays at home engaged in their repetitive activities, or watching the same videos, or doing nothing. The longer this goes on, the less likely the person concerned will want to lead a more active life. A small number may come to dominate the life of the family in the way described previously in this chapter. These situations arise be-cause of the lack of day and residential services suitable for more-able people with autistic disorders. Parents in this situation may find support and help from the Autism Society of America, which offers general information on employment for adults with autism as well as some relevant book references.

For adults who are unable to work or live independently, the best solution is residential accommodation in a home specifically for more-able people with autistic disorders. However, adults in this group can be found in every possible kind of sheltered accommodation, suitable or unsuitable. Some can be found among those living on the streets. Most who are unsuitably placed have never been diagnosed, so that it was never possible to make sensible plans for their future while they were children.

Employment

Appropriate employment that makes use of special skills and is enjoyed is the best way to maximize self-esteem and minimize disturbed behavior. More-able adults with autistic disorders are employed in a wide range of paid occupations. In addition to level of ability and area of special skill, certain factors are important for success. A sympathetic and knowledgeable employer and tolerant co-workers are among the essentials. Social and communication impairments exclude work that involves much interacting and talking with people. The lack of flexibility in an autistic person's make-up means that work where instructions are complicated and methods change frequently is likely to be unsuitable. Some adults may still be sensitive to noises and bright lights and may be unable to tolerate such conditions in a workplace. They tend to get upset if people are impatient or irritable or if anyone shouts loudly. When they start work they need someone to explain every little detail, to show them the cloakroom and toilets, how to collect lunch from the cafeteria, what time to start work and, equally important, when to stop. Someone needs to keep a watchful eye on them to make sure everything goes smoothly. Even the journey to work may have unexpected snags. With public transportation there is the risk that the usual bus or train may be late or cancelled and this may produce confusion and distress.

Those who can fit into open employment tend to be hardworking and conscientious. Once they have learned the rules they apply them with meticulous accuracy, although this can have its negative side, since striving for perfect accuracy may slow the work down to a level that is unacceptable. They are usually honest and without guile. If things go well, they are often popular with their colleagues once their disabilities are understood and accepted. Problems arise when employers and co-workers are not aware of the nature of the individual's specific impairments.

There are some among the more-able adults who, despite their skills, are unable to cope with employment, often because they are too rigid and repetitive to fit in with the demands of paid work. They require "sheltered" employment of the kind and in the conditions that are right for them. There are few specialized centers to cater for this group. Dependent upon the strengths and weaknesses of a given individual, day centers for people with learning difficulties may not to be able to provide for or to cope with those with autistic disorders, especially those who are more able, unless they have some staff with relevant training and experience and can make special provisions.

Marriage

One of the questions often asked by parents of young children with autistic disorders is "Will he/she ever marry and have children?" To date, follow-up studies of people who have been diagnosed in childhood as having autistic disorders show that virtually none of them marry. This is to be expected, given the severe social impairments.

The adults who may marry are those who have the triad of impairments in the most subtle form, are of average or high ability and, in most cases, have never been diagnosed as having an autistic disorder. Such marriages can work well if the partner values the person with the autistic disorder for their positive qualities and knows and accepts their eccentricities. When things go wrong, this is often because the partner wants empathy and emotional support, which the person with the autistic disorder cannot give.

Another source of difficulty is the autistic insistence on following a routine in the home that cannot be changed whatever the circumstances. Among the wives of men with autistic traits, there are some who seek help because of the stress of their everyday lives. In most cases they married without awareness of the problems ahead, or else thought that their influence would change their husbands. It is not possible to change anyone's character and behavior pattern, least of all someone with autistic traits. After a varying length of time they realize this and do not know what to do. In effect, there are only two courses of action. One is to accept the partner as they are and cope as well as possible; the other is to end the marriage or partnership. These are stark choices, especially if children are involved, but it is better to face the truth.

The advent of children may make things worse because their demands increase the need for mutual support between parents. Furthermore, babies and toddlers disrupt any attempts at an orderly life. As already mentioned there is good evidence of genetic factors in the cause of autistic disorders. The figures that are available to date concern the risk to parents of having a second child with an autistic disorder if they already have one. There are no statistics concerning the risks if one or both parents have an autistic disorder or have social or communication impairments or repetitive behavior in a subtle form, but research in the area of family genetics is ongoing and preliminary data seems to suggest that the risks are higher than for the general population.

Psychiatric Illness

Psychiatric illnesses can complicate autistic disorders in adolescence or adult life. They are diagnosed mainly in those who are more able and can thus give some account of symptoms.

The condition that occurs most often is depression. This tends to be associated with the development of some insight and recognition of being different from peers. Lack of friends, especially girl or boy friends, or failures at such relationships are frequent causes of depression. In many, probably the majority, the symptoms are relatively mild and are reactive to specific problems. Sometimes, however, the depression is severe, affecting appetite, sleep and general level of activity. Psychiatric treatment, including anti-depressants, may be needed in such cases. Counseling from someone who understands and is experienced with people with autistic disorders can be most helpful for the more-able adolescents and adults who are unhappy and finding it difficult to come to terms with their disabilities.

Other diagnosable psychiatric illnesses are less common. Episodes of mania or hypomania, or cycles of mania and depression can occur and require the appropriate treatment. The diagnosis of schizophrenia is particularly difficult to make in someone with an autistic disorder. The "negative" symptoms, such as lack of social interaction, paucity of speech and non-verbal communication, and lack of motivation, are common in both conditions. The "positive" symptoms of schizophrenia, that is the auditory hallucinations and delusional experiences, are difficult or impossible to describe for someone with the communication impairments of autistic disorders. Most people with autistic disorders, even those with good grammar and large vocabularies, have problems in understanding the meaning of questions to elicit the subjective experiences typical of schizophrenia. When confused and not knowing how to reply, they may say yes to anything.

A young man who worked in an office became agitated when he had to use a different room at work while his own was being painted. His behavior was so disturbed that he was admitted to a psychiatric unit. He had never previously been diagnosed as having an autistic disorder. He was asked if he heard voices when no one was in the room with him, to which he replied that he had just had this experience. Schizophrenia was suspected until it was discovered that he was referring to the fact that he could overhear speakers in the next room through the thin partition. On taking a history from his parents, an autistic disorder of the Asperger type was diagnosed.

Much care is needed before concluding that schizophrenia is present but if such an illness does occur in someone with an autistic disorder it should be treated appropriately, including giving the most effective medication.

This story illustrates another aspect of the psychiatric complications of autistic disorders. When under stress, even a previously able and comparatively well-adjusted adolescent or young adult can become disturbed in behavior with rambling and incoherent speech. Actions can appear to be random and wildly inappropriate. The term "psychotic" is often used for such states but adds nothing to one's understanding of them. They are not the same as schizophrenia though there may be non-specific delusions and hallucinations and odd perceptual experiences. The problems usually disappear if the source of stress can be identified and removed.

In a few adolescents or young adults, the repetitive routines of childhood develop into behavior like that seen in obsessive compulsive disorders. This may take the form of constant hand washing, or insistence on performing certain actions, such as doing up buttons in a precise way and starting again if any errors are made, or thinking the same thoughts repetitively. Phobias such as fear of germs can become intense and be accompanied by repetitive rituals to prevent contamination. This raises interesting questions concerning the relationship between autistic disorders and obsessive-compulsive states. The medication that has been found helpful in treating obsessive-compulsive states may be effective for this type of behavior in people with autistic disorders.

A very small proportion of adolescents and young adults gradually become slower and slower in their actions. They may become fixed in postures, perhaps with a spoon of food halfway to their mouths, and stay in this state for some seconds, minutes or even longer. They may have difficulty in crossing thresholds between rooms or demarcations between two types of flooring, taking tiny steps forward and then back, over and over again. They may be unable to initiate any action, such as rising from a chair, unless prompted by seeing someone else do this. They may cease speaking and lose all initiative, including not going to the toilet so that bladder and bowels fill to overflowing. This is called catatonia. It seems to be an inability to make an effort of will to initiate a movement. It is just like the catatonic states that followed the epidemic of *encephalitis lethargica* that occurred during and after World War I and that were shown in the film of Oliver Sacks' book on the subject, *Awakenings*. In some cases, this state is reached after the individual has gone through the stage of developing obsessive-compulsive behavior. The repetitive rituals take longer and longer and the movements become slower and slower until finally the person is in a catatonic state.

In people in catatonic states, the automatic patterns of movement that were learned before the catatonia started can still be carried on as long as the individual is helped to begin. Actions such as riding a bicycle, jumping on a trampoline or returning a football may be possible. Also, moving along a well-defined path is easier than crossing open unmarked ground. These facts give a guide for helping those affected. They must not be left to sit idle but should be prompted through all the activities of each day. They should be encouraged to engage in all the automatic sequences of movement they developed prior to the catatonia. It should be noted that it may be as hard for the person concerned to stop such movements once started as it was to start them in the first place. The activities should be monitored so that they are not carried on to the point of exhaustion. It has been reported that anti-depressants has proved helpful in some cases of catatonia but the effects of medication are variable and prescribing is a matter of trial and error.

Catatonia can occur in adolescents and young adults with autistic disorders of any level of ability. The reasons why it happens are not known, neither is there any work on what proportion of individuals are affected, although it is clear that the numbers are very small.

For all psychiatric illnesses that complicate autistic conditions, the appropriate treatment should be given. However, the underlying autistic disorder must not be overlooked. The special needs resulting from this long-term disability remain, even if the psychiatric complication is successfully treated. Ideally, adult as well as child psychiatrists should have training and experience with autistic disorders because they will meet people with these disabilities in all areas of their clinical work. They should be aware of the services they need so that they can refer them on to the relevant agencies for long-term help.

Delinquent and Criminal Behavior

Adolescents and adults with autistic disorders who have mild learning difficulties or borderline, average or high levels of ability may commit acts that bring them into conflict with the law. This only happens to a small minority. The majority are extremely law-abiding because they are concerned with following the rules in every tiny detail.

There are various reasons why a few break the law. Some are unaware that particular laws apply to them and cannot understand what all the fuss is about. One young man took money from his aunt's house because he thought it would buy him some friends. He found it in a drawer, not her handbag, so innocently assumed he could take it.

The pursuit of special interests can lead to trouble. An adolescent girl was fascinated by the characteristics of different breeds of dogs, though she had no liking for real dogs. She took some books on dogs from a bookstore without paying. She did this twice without being detected but on the third occasion she was caught. She was indignant because she thought that the fact that no one stopped her on the first two occasions demonstrated that she was allowed to take the books she wanted. Her evident oddness and guileless innocence saved her from prosecution.

In a small number of cases, the social impairment takes the form of total indifference to other people. If this is allied to a special interest in, for example, weapons or chemicals, there may be the temptation to try the effects on someone.

Paranoid feelings may be particularly strong in a few individuals, often based on real experiences of rejection or teasing by age peers. The desire for revenge can lead to physical aggression, attacks on property, or some other illegal act. Parents may be the object of such attacks if they are undeservedly blamed for the individual's problems.

Occasionally, a teenage boy attaches himself to a group of age peers who engage in delinquency. The young person with the autistic disorder follows the gang because it is the nearest approach to friendship he can find. It is likely that, sooner or later, he will be the one member of the gang who is caught while the others are quick enough to run away.

As already emphasized, the proportion of autistic people who carry out delinquent or criminal acts is very small. If the diagnosis is made in early childhood and appropriate education and a structured, organized program are provided, the chances of illegal behavior occurring in adolescence or adult life are minimized. If such problems do occur, or seem likely, parents should seek help from psychiatric and social services. As mentioned before, it is of no help to anyone, least of all to the young person with an autistic disorder, to try to hide the problems.

The Borderlines with Normalcy

Many of the features that are characteristic of autistic disorders can be found to a lesser degree in individuals who are functioning well in all aspects of life. Most people can identify one or more aspects of their own personalities that have something in common with autistic behavior. As Asperger pointed out, some degree of autism is an advantage for those in the fields of art or science.

There is no clear cut-off point between autistic disorders in the most-able people and what might be called eccentric normality. In discussions on problems of diagnosis it is often asked where the line should be drawn. Is there not a danger of harming someone by giving them a diagnosis and causing problems that did not exist before? This is a theoretical rather than a practical dilemma. In clinical work, the primary reason for making a diagnosis of an autistic disorder is that the individuals concerned are experiencing major difficulties in development from infancy to adult life and their parents, or occasionally the persons themselves, are asking for help.

In these circumstances it is appropriate to investigate in order to make a diagnosis from which recommendations can follow. Individuals who are coping well, even if they have many autistic traits, will not be referred or refer themselves for diagnosis and it would be an unwarranted interference to suggest that they should. A group of very able people who are aware that they have an autistic disorder and who keep in touch with each other have made the point in various publications that their way of thinking and experiencing the world is valid for them and they would not want to be "cured" even if this were possible. Of course, not all those with insight feel this way and some do ask for help even though they are, ostensibly, coping well. The feelings and wishes of each individual should be respected.

PART III

Ways of Helping

CHAPTER 16

Services

In this chapter I'll discuss the roles of different kinds of professionals and the services they offer in relation to autistic disorders. The aim is to give parents some idea of where to begin looking for the help they need for their child and to address some of the concerns of professional workers in the field of autism.

How well or how badly a visit to any professional worker goes depends not only on the child or adult concerned, but on the knowledge, experience, and attitude of the professional involved, as well as their assistants and receptionists. Should parents encounter a professional who is unfamiliar with autism, the parents or other caregivers need to explain as much as they can about the disability and suggest ways of approaching the autistic person. Most professionals are interested and willing to help. However, if a parent is unfortunate enough to meet one of the minority who are impatient or hostile, I would suggest following up the visit with a letter couched in positive terms to the appropriate person explaining autism and suggesting how things could be managed better in the future. It might be helpful if this was accompanied by a letter and some general information from a local autistic group, perhaps inviting the professional and coworkers to a workshop about autism. No opportunity for education should be lost.

Assessment

The diagnosis of an autistic disorder may first be suspected by the parents or by a variety of professionals in touch with the child, such as pediatricians, teachers, or speech therapists. In the case of adults who have never been diagnosed in childhood, a psychiatrist for adult illnesses, a social worker, or a residential care worker may be the first to suspect an autistic condition. Because Asperger syndrome was only added to the DSM-IV within the last decade, sometimes the first suspicions that a given adult fits this classification may originate with a family member who has read relevant information, or even with the individual himself. For children, the first referral to confirm the diagnosis is usually to the local pediatrician, child psychiatrist or psychologist, or child guidance clinic. Parents may find all the information and help they need through these local resources. If not, they have a right to ask for a second opinion.

There are currently a small number of centers in the United States that specialize in the diagnosis and assessment of children and adolescents with social and communication disorders. Parents and caregivers should be aware that these centers are usually in high demand and often have lengthy wait lists. The fee for an evaluation may be quite high, and parents should be sure to clarify payment options prior to scheduling an appointment, as not all autism centers accept insurance. Access to autism centers varies widely across the country, and because the field of autism is a growing area, new facilities may emerge in areas that were previously lacking in resources. In general, centers are more frequently located in major cities and are most often affiliated with hospitals and universities. The best way to keep abreast of changing services is through national organizations such as the Autism Society of America and the Asperger Syndrome Coalition of the U.S. (ASC–US). These and other organizations offer general information about autism spectrum disorders, state-by-state resources, book titles, parent support groups, and training for professionals. The internet is also an excellent tool for accessing this information and is addressed in further detail at the end of the chapter.

Diagnosis and Medical Investigations

The first edition of this book carried the implicit assumption that diagnosis of autistic disorders was always made by a doctor; this is no longer the case. Now a number of clinical psychologists have made these disorders their special field and have developed expertise in diagnostic methods. It is still likely that medically qualified professionals, especially pediatricians and child psychiatrists, will be required to diagnose developmental disorders. Their knowledge is needed for medical investigations and the recognition of any associated physical conditions. Even more important than a professional's specific degree, however, is his or her level of knowledge and experience in the field of autism. Because autistic disorders involve deficits in a range of skills, children will benefit from assessment in a number of areas by a group of professionals working together. Ideally parents should seek a multidisciplinary evaluation that is conducted by a team of professionals with experience and expertise in the field of autism. Such a team might consist of a pediatrician, psychiatrist, psychologist, speech and language pathologist, and physical therapist, or a similar combination of professionals.

Over the last three decades the school of thought that denies the reality of mental illness and disability has influenced some parents and others. Some people are opposed to "labeling" a person. Those who hold these views believe that giving a name to a condition is a self-fulfilling prophesy that harms the person concerned. In reality, having an accurate and detailed diagnosis as early as possible is the first crucial step for parents. A diagnosis enables parents to find information and help and gives them access to services and to the support found from meeting other parents in the same situation. Although it is intensely distressing to know that your child has a serious developmental disability, most parents are relieved to have an explanation for their child's puzzling behavior. It also affords them the possibility of following a plan of action. In response to the anti-labeling theory, one parent pointed out that children with odd behavior cannot avoid labels of some kind; she would rather have the child correctly diagnosed as autistic than labeled "that spoiled child with awful behavior." It should be noted that in some cases, for instance if the child is very young, a definitive diagnosis may not initially be possible. A detailed description of the child's difficulties and solid recommendations for intervention are as important as the diagnosis itself.

A full diagnostic evaluation involves taking a detailed developmental history, psychological assessment, observation of behavior, examination for any additional medical or psychiatric conditions and disabilities (including hearing or vision impairments), and investigations to try establishing the original cause of the disability. With regard to establishing the cause, there are some differences of opinion. In Sweden, for example, a full medical work-up is carried out for all children referred to clinics for developmental disorders, including tests of blood and cerebro-spinal fluid. These tests ensure that no associated conditions are missed; they are informative for the parents and are of value for research in this area. In the U.S. the investigations are generally much less extensive unless clear clinical indications suggest that particular tests should be done. This is because detailed investigations rarely show abnormalities that are relevant for treatment, they can be distressing for the child, and they are expensive. However, standard diagnostic procedure may vary depending on the policies of a particular hospital or clinic.

Health and Social Services

Family Doctors

Despite the increased awareness of autistic disorders, many parents still have problems finding the proper diagnosis for their child. Recognizing autistic disorders requires knowledge and experience. Since the autistic spectrum is relatively uncommon when compared with other physical illnesses, most family doctors are unfamiliar with these conditions. Doctors in general practice are much more familiar with physical symptoms and signs than with the unusual behavior of an autistic child who looks alert, attractive and physically healthy. Even for professionals with experience, it is necessary to be cautious when diagnosing children under five years of age. Differentiating between various autism spectrum disorders such as autism, Asperger syndrome, and PDD-NOS can be particularly challenging when children are young. Behavior and other symptoms can change substantially later, particularly around five to six years when children may be beginning school and are asked to adjust to new routines and larger peer groups. Language gains can affect the diagnostic picture; early intervention may also alter the way a child presents symptoms.

The family doctor is often the first person to be approached by parents when they are concerned that something is wrong. Even though most family doctors are not experts in recognizing autistic disorders, they can listen to the parents' concerns and refer them to a specialist in the field of developmental disorders. Family doctors should avoid the three most unhelpful statements that can be made to a mother who is worried about her child's development: "You are an overanxious mother"; "He/she will grow out of it"; and "It must be the way you are bringing her/him up."

TREATMENT OF PHYSICAL ILLNESSES AND DISABILITIES

A child with an autistic disorder may also have any other type of physical disability or illness. Generally, the more disabilities a child has, the harder it is to cope with life. It is therefore important to make sure a child with an autistic disorder is as physically fit as possible and to give whatever therapeutic treatment is necessary. A diagnosis of any illness can be difficult because lower-functioning people with autism often do not complain and cannot describe their symptoms. Information from parents or caregivers, who know the person better than anyone else, may offer the best clues as to what is wrong.

Routine physical care, such as inoculations and treatment for physical illnesses, can be a problem because many children with autism have intense resistance to any interference. They dislike the change in routine, hate being touched, and are disturbed by the unfamiliar smells, sights, and sounds of a medical surrounding. However, some children and adults with autistic disorders actually like having medical attention. Some are indifferent to pain and are fascinated by the technical details of the procedures. Others seem to enjoy being the center of so much attention and sympathy without having to do anything. As with all disabled children, family doctors can do their work more effectively if they get to know the child and establish a sense of trust before any medical attention is needed.

Having to wait a long time to be seen by a physician is a strain on any child, particularly for those with autistic disorders who have no idea why they are in a strange place for so long. It is also hard on the parents and the other patients if the child's behavior becomes disturbed. If possible, the receptionist should be informed ahead of time and an understanding doctor should try to arrange appointments to avoid this problem.

Clinical Psychologists

Often psychologists are involved in diagnosing the presence of autistic spectrum disorders. Their specific role in the diagnostic process is assessment of the individual's pattern of abilities and disabilities. Standardized psychological tests of many kinds, together with observation of the child's behavior in structured and unstructured situations, are used in this process. When the information obtained in this way is put together with the details of the developmental history, the behavior in different settings and the medical findings, a complete diagnostic formulation can be made. This is of great value for helping parents understand their child and as a basis for planning education.

Psychologists have also made a major contribution to helping children and adults with autistic disorders by developing methods of behavior management that emphasize organizing the living environment of the affected person. Some of the original ideas in this area have had to be modified or discarded, but much has been learned over the years and the environmental/behavioral approach to behavior problems is still the most effective method currently available. Clinical psychologists provide services for both children and adults in the areas of learning difficulties, social skills training, and psychiatric conditions. Some work privately and others may do sessions in schools, homes, or daycare centers where there are people with autistic disorders.

Counselors

People whose original training is in psychology, psychiatry, social work, or other professions may be involved in counseling either individuals with autistic disorders, their parents and families, or both.

Sometimes higher-functioning adolescents and adults with autistic disorders, who are able to talk fairly well and who have made good progress, become unhappily aware that they are different from others in their age group. This occurs most frequently with individuals who have Asperger syndrome. Such people may be helped by sensible and sensitive counseling from psychologists or other professional workers who understand the nature of their disabilities.

As with anyone, individuals with autistic disorders can become depressed by the loss of someone they love and depend on or by other major life crises, and may need the help of an experienced counselor at these times. Some autistic people with good abilities who are trying to live independently rely on ready access to practical advice and emotional support from a counselor they like and trust.

Practical counseling, based on understanding of the nature of autistic disorders and solid common sense, is different from psychotherapy and psychoanalysis based on theoretical concepts of the human psyche. These latter two methods have been attempted with children and adults with autistic disorders, but there is no evidence that they are effective in curing or even diminishing the person's disabilities. Psychotherapeutic techniques that presuppose the development of complex language and the ability to introspect and understand symbolic ideas are particularly inappropriate. The interpretations given by the therapist are liable to confuse individuals with autistic disorders and to implant bizarre ideas, which they may talk about on the most unsuitable occasions. Play therapy is equally pointless in children with impairments of imaginative development.

While some families find they can accept a disabled child fairly easily and come to terms with their unhappiness as time goes on, others are less philosophical for a variety of personal reasons. Many would be helped by counseling from an experienced professional who understands what it is like to have a child with a developmental disability. Such counseling can help diminish any tendency to blame oneself and to release the parents' energies for more constructive activities in relation to their child. The times when support from an experienced counselor are particularly needed are when the diagnosis of an autistic disorder is first made, when the child is approaching school age, on starting school, when the child reaches adolescence, at school-leaving, and at the time of admission to long-term residential care.

Professional workers who hold theories implying that the parents cause their child to become autistic may recommend that these parents undergo psychotherapy or psychoanalysis in order to help the child indirectly. There is no evidence that these methods are useful. Insofar as they exacerbate self-blame, they only do harm.

Treatment for Psychiatric Disorders for Adults with Autism

Psychiatrists for adult psychiatric conditions or for learning difficulties may be called on to treat adults who have psychiatric illnesses associated with autistic disorders. There are no specialist services for people with autistic disorders who develop psychiatric illnesses. Such persons are treated as out- or inpatients by psychiatrists who treat people with psychiatric conditions or by psychiatrists who treat those with learning difficulties. However, a psychiatrist's level of familiarity with autism can make a significant difference in treatment, and whenever possible a psychiatrist with a specialty in autism should be selected.

Admission to a hospital ward for adult psychiatric illness or for people who have learning difficulties and disturbed behavior can be a traumatic experience for someone with an autistic disorder. The illnesses of the other residents mean that events are unpredictable, at times chaotic, which is the worst possible environment for someone with an autistic disorder. Treatment within the individual's own familiar environment, with medication if necessary, given by a psychiatrist who is familiar with autistic disorders, is the best solution when possible. Sometimes admission to a hospital is essential. If the entire staff in a psychiatric establishment is given some training in the nature of autistic disorders and the needs of the people concerned, they will be better- equipped to reduce problems, since they will, no doubt, have to work with people who have these conditions.

Some adults with autistic disorders who commit serious crimes as a result of their lack of understanding of social rules are sent to prison if the diagnosis is not recognized. Others are placed in secure mental facilities. Awareness of autistic disorders is growing among correctional officers and hospital staff, and some police forces and hospitals are now offering their staff workshops and specialized training in dealing with children and adults who have autistic disorders. However, levels of knowledge and awareness still vary widely among professionals, and there are many who have had no formal training or experience in this area.

Social Services

Social workers include those employed by schools, government agencies, hospitals, clinics and volunteer groups, and those who work privately. They have two primary roles. One is helping families obtain the kinds of services and benefits they need and to which they are entitled, and the other is to provide counseling for individuals and families.

Social services for people with autistic disorders vary from state to state. All we can do here is mention some of the functions that may be relevant for people with autistic disorders and their families. Parents should make direct inquiries to see if help for any particular problem is available, even if it is not mentioned in the following brief list.

The type of social services available will vary depending on the characteristics of the individual, such as age (child or adult) and the nature of the disability (e.g., the specific diagnosis, mental retardation status). Social workers or parent advocates can be helpful in informing parents of their legal rights and helping them obtain services. In some extreme cases, hiring a lawyer may be necessary to procure services to which individuals are legally entitled. Demand for services typically exceeds what is available, and state social services, with constraints on their budgets, often have little time available for individual and family counseling. Social workers employed by other agencies or working privately can give this kind of help, but again, these resources are limited and those who are experienced with autistic disorders are few and far between.

One of the roles of social workers is to support families in their dealings with educational, health and voluntary and private institutions, and to coordinate the work of all these agencies.

It is useful for parents to inform local social service agencies that they have a child with a disability *before* they are in need of help. Not only is the system overloaded, but it can also take time to wade through bureaucracy; those running the services are likely to be able to foresee future demands if they're prepared. Social workers can provide advice on the complex system of financial benefits that people with disabilities and their caregivers are entitled to, and can often help families obtain them.

Social workers can also help find a range of relevant day and residential services for adults and for the provision of respite care, practical help in the home, and various kinds of equipment for use in the home. They may be able to help parents with travel to specialist facilities and arrangements for the provision of meals, as well as having a role in the care and protection of children. Social workers should also be a source of information about voluntary groups of all kinds that provide helpful services.

Dental Services

Teeth cleaning can be a major problem for children with autistic disorders. They may be unable or unwilling to clean their own teeth and resist when their parents try. They may eat only soft or sweet foods and demand large quantities of drinks that are bad for the teeth. Gum disease, dental decay, toothache, and even a dental abscess can occur without any sign from the child that something is wrong. Sometimes the child's behavior becomes disturbed in response to a painful condition, but they are unable to indicate the site of the problem.

Regular dental care is essential but may be hard to organize if the child refuses to cooperate. There are some dentists with a special interest in treating children or adults with learning difficulties, including autistic disorders. Some have special experience because they provide a service for a school, residential home, or hospital that caters to children or adults with autistic disorders. Some have developed special techniques for gaining trust and cooperation, even from children with severe autistic disorders. It often takes a long time before any treatment can be given, but time taken beforehand to get to know the child is well spent. Interestingly, in some cases, after intense resistance a child switches and enjoys visits to the dentist. This is one of the many paradoxes presented by children with autistic disorders.

We are unaware of special dental services solely for children or adults with autistic disorders. Parents can find out about dentists in their own area with special expertise in autistic disorders by making inquiries to other parents of autistic children, local autism support groups, and relevant local services, such as those for people with learning difficulties.

Other Therapists

Physiotherapy and a program of physical exercises can be helpful with the common problems of motor coordination, especially organizing movements in relation to other people.

The skills of physical and occupational therapists are valuable in devising and teaching motor skills and constructive activities. Teachers and instructors who can engage the children or adults in physical education and other physical pursuits of all kinds, including horseback riding and swimming, are much needed because of the positive effects of these activities. Motor skills are often an area of weakness in individuals with Asperger syndrome and regular work with a physical or occupational therapist is an important component of intervention.

Some music therapists are very interested in working with children or adults with autistic disorders because many of these children and adults are more responsive to music than to speech.

Aromatherapy, massage and techniques for encouraging relaxation, dance and drama are much enjoyed by many people with autistic disorders of all ages and may help to reduce tension and disturbed behavior.

These types of specialists can make a valuable contribution as members of a team of therapists working with people who have autistic disorders. Difficulties arise, however, if any one specialist assumes that they alone can help or cure the condition. Another common misconception is the therapist believing that what he or she is treating is the cause of the whole clinical picture. One example mentioned earlier is the "semantic-pragmatic language disorder," which has been used as a diagnostic category, preventing recognition of an autistic disorder in higher-functioning children with fluent speech (see Chapter 5). Another is the theory that the lack of integration of different kinds of sensory input is the basis of autistic behavior, or even a separate diagnostic category. These ideas arise when the therapists concerned do not take into account the whole history and clinical picture.

Advocates of "Curative Treatments"

Every condition that produces lifelong disabilities and for which there is no effective treatment has been the focus of claims for curative methods. Autistic disorders are no exception. The so-called cures have included medications, diets, psychotherapies, behavior therapies and methods that might be described as mystical or magical. Some methods have come and gone, only to return under another name or in another form. It must be emphasized here that educational methods that have proven their worth in practice do not cure children of their autistic disorders. They facilitate the development of potential skills a person may have. There is a close analogy with education for children who have visual or hearing impairments. Education teaches them skills but does not cure their biological disabilities.

There are three main problems in evaluating any possible claims that a treatment is curative. First, almost all methods, except for the most bizarre, tend to have a grain of truth in them. For example, holding and cuddling a child through a temper tantrum can be helpful, and holding accustoms the child to being held, but this does not mean the basic impairments have been cured. Teaching practical skills by guiding a child's limbs is a useful technique, but not a justification for claims made that "facilitated communication" cures autism. "Auditory integration therapy" may reduce oversensitivity to sound but there is no objective evidence that it does anything else. Second, children with autistic disorders go through phases of more and less difficult behavior and tend to develop skills in sudden spurts. If a good phase or acquiring a new skill coincides by chance with a new "treatment," the treatment could be credited with the improvement. Third, any outcome in adult life is closely linked to the innate level of ability. Those with high levels of skill are likely to do well as long as they are educated appropriately no matter what "treatment" they receive. Therapists who select the most able children for their special treatment are bound to have apparent successes.

Proper evaluation requires carefully organized and controlled trials done by objective observers who are not involved in any way with the advocates of the treatments. There must be adequate methods of measuring any changes, and longterm followup assessment of any later consequences of the method. The few methods that have received proper testing have been shown not to have the effects claimed.

Of course, parents do have the right to try any treatment that is not potentially harmful and is ethically acceptable. They should, however, beware of those who play on parents' feelings of guilt and despair and their desire to clutch at any straw. The Autism Society of America offers information concerning various "treatments" to date but does not advocate any of them.

Education

School Psychologists

Research and practical experience has shown that the right kind of education is crucial for the development of autistic children's full potential. School psychologists are concerned with assessment of children who are having learning difficulties in the classroom. Their role also includes advising teachers on special educational programs for such children. In order for a child to have special educational help, his or her needs have to be formally recognized. Children who are suspected of having a disability are generally given a comprehensive assessment. This assessment may be conducted by an individual school psychologist or by the school team, which may include a psychologist, a speech and language pathologist, a physical or occupational therapist, and teachers. At a minimum, evaluations generally involve cognitive (IQ) testing, a parent interview and a general overview of the child's behaviors as observed by the psychologist. More comprehensive evaluations also include teacher interviews, classroom observations, speech and language testing, an evaluation of muscle and motor coordination and specific testing for suspected problem areas such as attentional difficulties, memory deficits, processing difficulties, social-emotional concerns and a variety of other areas. After completing an evaluation of their own, the team may occasionally feel that an outside evaluation is warranted. In this case the cost of an evaluation by a professional outside of the educational system may be covered by the school.

Teachers

Teachers have the burden of putting all the recommendations into effect in the classroom. They also have to work closely together with parents and other professionals involved. They need training, experience, and sympathetic understanding of the children. Together with parents, caregivers in residential establishments and teachers have the most demanding roles of anyone involved with people who have autistic disorders.

Speech and Language Therapists

Language problems are, by definition, intrinsic to autistic disorders, but the fundamental impairments affect the way language is used for communication, not just the structure of language. Therapists who are interested in enhancing social and communication skills, including comprehension and use of all methods of communicating, have a valuable contribution to make. They may be the first to suspect that a child with a language problem has an autistic disorder and can contribute to the diagnostic assessment. In schools, they can work directly with autistic children and guide teachers and parents in ways of enhancing the children's social and communication skills.

Language therapists who are of most help are those who are concerned with a child's whole pattern of behavior, not solely with language. Too narrow a view of language therapy that ignores the rest of the child's behavior can lead to the assumption that the language problem exists in isolation, thus denying any underlying autistic disorder.

Speech and language therapists work in a variety of settings including both public and private schools, clinics, residential programs and private practices. Some specialize in a specific aspect of speech or language, such as articulation, or work with a specific population, such as children with autism and other pervasive developmental disorders. While the majority of speech and language therapists work with children, some specialize in working with adults.

Preschool Services

Research has shown that early intervention has a significant impact on the eventual outcome for individuals with autistic spectrum disorders. State-run "Birth to Three" programs ensure that children under the age of three receive the early intervention they are legally entitled to. The amount and type of intervention a child receives varies widely, however. Parents should contact their state program immediately after receiving a diagnosis or as soon as they suspect their young child may have a disability. For contact information, see "The Internet as a Resource," below.

Many young children with autistic disorders benefit from attending some kind of preschool group, and often playgroups or nursery schools will accept children with disabilities. Some cater specifically to young children with disabilities. Even if, as usually happens, the child with an autistic disorder does not voluntarily mix with the other children, he or she gradually becomes accustomed to the proximity of age peers. At first, they may be distressed by being in a group, or react with aggression to children who approach them. This can usually be overcome if they are initially allowed to be on their own, away from the others, while a relationship with the staff is developed. They can then be led by an adult they trust into closer contact with the other children. At this preschool stage, mixing with children without disabilities often works well. There is no pressure to engage in tasks beyond the child's capacity and very young children have not yet developed the strong group feeling that can at a later age lead to rejection of those who are different. It should be noted, however, that children with autism usually benefit from small groups or one-to-one aides in the preschool setting and may require additional one-on-one teaching of basic skills from professionals who may work with the child at home.

When there is a choice between a specialized program for toddlers with developmental delays of all kinds and an ordinary playgroup or nursery school, the decision must depend upon the individual child and his specific needs. The most important factor for young children is that early and intensive intervention should be sought.

Educational Services

All types of school—special and mainstream, public and private—have accepted children with autistic disorders. Some further education colleges also cater to their special needs.

There are a small number of private residential and day schools across the U.S. that focus on special education. Few are exclusively for individuals with autistic spectrum disorders, but rather accept children with a range of learning disabilities or even social and emotional difficulties. Areas of emphasis also range. Some focus primarily on academics, while others are more concerned with teaching social skills or independent living skills. These private schools are often extremely costly and may or may not offer financial assistance. Specialized schools are not always the best option for an individual with autism. Some children are better served in traditional public schools in special education programs or in mainstream classrooms. The best placement will depend on the skills and needs of an individual child. Some schools, public or private, offer an extended school year program. Often autistic children will benefit from a school program that extends through the summer as this is a time when skills can easily be lost.

To Mainstream or Attend a Special School?

There is currently a dispute concerning education for children with disabilities. Pressure from some quarters advocates education in mainstream schools for every child, regardless of the nature of their disability, in order to ensure equality of opportunity and to avoid the stigma of segregation. There is no doubt that very many, perhaps most, children with disabilities benefit from mainstream schooling with their age peers. However, the desire to include in mainstream education all children with specific or general learning difficulties is based on theory rather than on the knowledge and understanding of each individual child's real needs.

With regard to children with autistic disorders, the situation is complicated because they vary so widely in their levels of ability and their patterns of behavior. It is often argued that all children need normal role models, especially for developing social skills. It is suggested that autistic children cannot become sociable if they are educated together with other children who are equally socially impaired. There are some children among the more able who do well in mainstream schools, especially in some small private schools that will take children with academic ability who have special needs. Some autistic children have enough insight to try to learn social rules by observing other children, though they make many mistakes and would benefit from specific teaching of social skills.

However, the majority of children with autistic disorders, because of the nature of their impairments, do not learn by copying their age peers. They learn social skills by rote if specifically taught by adults who are experienced in appropriate teaching techniques. Apart from those with good academic ability, the children's pace and methods of learning differ markedly from those of other children, making it difficult for teachers to cope with such a diversity of need. This point is discussed in detail in the book by Rita Jordan and Stuart Powell, *Understanding and Teaching Children with Autism*. If the child has a non-teaching assistant he or she may be able to integrate successfully but if he cannot join in any of the lessons and has to be involved with special activities in class and playtime there seems no point in continuing with mainstream education for the sake of an ideal.

The other major problem faced in mainstreaming is the attitude of other children. This has already been mentioned in Chapter 15, but it is important enough to merit repetition in this context. Whereas young children usually accept those who are different, older children and adolescents tend to apply strong pressures to conform to group norms and are intolerant of those who do not fit in. This can lead to teasing and bullying if the child who is different is not protected by adult supervision. Much of this persecution occurs on the playground or before or after school, unobserved by the staff. The child concerned, because of communication impairments, may never tell parents or teachers while suffering in silence. If the child has never been diagnosed, teachers may be irritated by their stubbornness and lack of respect for those with authority and may be unsympathetic or even blame the child for any disturbance in the class. Some children have been desperately unhappy in a mainstream school, developing reactive depression or other psychiatric disorders in adolescence. In my clinical experience, some adults carry the memory of miserable school days with them always and a very few have tried to revenge themselves in inappropriate ways.

The most reasonable approach to this issue is to acknowledge that a range of types of schools is required and that each individual child's needs should be assessed before deciding on their placement. The child's progress and emotional adjustment in the school should be monitored and changes made if necessary. There are some more able children with autistic disorders who can hold their own in mainstream schools and mainstream classrooms. They have made up their own minds that this is the type of education they want despite all the difficulties. Such children should be given every help and encouragement to stay in the school and class of their choice. Those who cannot cope, especially if they are unhappy, should be placed in special schools. This should not be regarded as an all-or-nothing decision.

It works well if a mainstream school and a special school cooperate so that children from the latter can attend specific sessions with the mainstream children when appropriate. They may eventually achieve full integration, but this should not be forced if it is not in the child's best interests. Ideally, if there is a partnership between a mainstream and a special school, the mainstream children spend some time in the special school in order to broaden their understanding of disabilities, as well as to help the children with special needs.

Types of Special Schools

Among the special schools or special classrooms, those designed for children with emotional and behavioral disturbance are the least likely to be suitable for children with autistic disorders. There are some exceptions in which the staff is able to provide for autistic children's special needs, but in most cases, the interests of the other children conflict too markedly with those who have autistic disorders. With the more able children there is also the possibility that they will learn, in a naive fashion, delinquent attitudes and activities from their schoolmates. More frequently, however, bullying is the main problem when autistic children are placed in settings of this kind.

Schools for children with learning disabilities or other clinical disorders tend to have larger proportions of children with autistic disorders among their pupils than other types of schools. This type of placement is appropriate for some of the children with autism, especially if the staff are interested in and have training in teaching children with autistic disorders and the school program is sufficiently structured and organized.

Parents of children who have typical autistic behavior with no physical signs of disability, but who have severe or profound learning difficulties, are often worried and confused when it is suggested that their child should attend a school for children with a wide range of disabilities. Many would prefer to have them educated in schools that specialize in autistic disorders. They are further distressed by the physical disabilities of many children in these schools. The fact is that there are few specialist schools available, and it is unlikely, to put it mildly, that there will ever be enough to cater to children with autistic disorders. The most sensible solution is for some staff in all schools that may take children with autistic disorders to undertake training in methods of teaching autistic spectrum children. It would be helpful for schools to experiment with different ways of organizing teaching for children with autistic disorders to see if special classes, special groups within classes, or some other system works best. Care has to be taken to ensure that resources are not removed from other children with special needs. Ideally, all the different specific impairments to be found among children with all kinds of developmental disorders should be analyzed and appropriately addressed in their educational programs. Teachers who understand the basic principles of teaching children with autistic disorders are in a better position to apply their knowledge to other disabilities. In areas where there are no schools with a special interest in autistic disorders, parents may be effective in bringing about change if they act together to apply pressure.

The few schools specializing in the education of children with autistic disorders are the pioneers in developing methods of teaching. They are most appropriate for children with potential skills who are unable to cope in other types of school, often because of their behavior. The most able children, including those who have the pattern of Asperger's syndrome, who are unhappy and not making progress in mainstream school, present a special problem. They might best be taught with the methods that suit other children with autistic disorders, but are too advanced in schoolwork to fit into most of the specialist schools. A very few schools are emerging that focus specifically on children with Asperger syndrome, such as the STAR Program in New York. However, limited programs and small classroom sizes mean that lengthy wait lists are the norm for such programs.

Unorthodox Educational Approaches

Claims have been made concerning the results of several unorthodox educational methods, including Daily Life Therapy at the Higashi schools in Boston and Tokyo; the Waldon approach; behavior modification as used by Ivar Lovaas; Feuerstein's Mediated Learning; Low Intrusion Teaching, Gentle Teaching and others. These programs have not been evaluated by independent research workers. There is much overlap among these methods and many similarities with more orthodox approaches. They do not have anything completely new to offer, although each has some useful ideas. The TEACCH approach developed in North Carolina is particularly valuable as a method of designing organized but individualized programs.

Educational Assessment

The educational rights of children with autism are governed by the Individuals with Disabilities Education Act (IDEA). Passed in 1975 and amended in 1997, this federal law states that all children in the United States have the right to a "free, appropriate public education in the least restrictive environment regardless of the level or severity of their disability." The law mandates that each child's specific educational placement be determined on an individual basis and placement with non-disabled children is sought to the maximum extent that is reasonable. School systems are responsible for providing multidisciplinary evaluations for children between the ages of three and twenty-one that assess all areas in which the child is suspected of having a disability. If the school is not able to offer an appropriate evaluation, or if parents are unhappy with the evaluation offered, parents have the right to seek a second evaluation outside of the school system. This evaluation must be honored by the school in planning for a child's curriculum. However, if the school can prove that their evaluation meets the criteria for appropriateness, parents may have to pay for this second evaluation themselves. Evaluations may be requested by the parents when they first suspect the child may have a disability. The school system may also determine that there is a need for evaluation; however, written parental consent is necessary before the evaluation commences. Reevaluations are required every three years (often referred to as "Triennial Reviews") and may also be requested when the child's level of functioning in one or more areas changes. The findings from the evaluations are then used to write an Individualized Education Program (IEP), which outlines the student's needs, the special education goals and the services that will be provided.

If parents are unhappy with the evaluation, the IEP or the delivery of services, several options are available. In discussions with the IEP team, parents can arrange for an advocate to help them represent their views. Referrals to advocates can generally be obtained through local autism societies or parent support groups. Mediation between the parents and the school system by a neutral third party is a second approach. If this effort is unsatisfactory, parents may take legal action via a due process hearing.

The needs of a child under three years of age are also addressed in the Individuals with Disabilities Education Act Amendments of 1997, which includes a special section on infants and toddlers with disabilities. Specific mandates apply to early intervention for these young children and services are generally offered through state-run "Birth to Three" programs. For older children, federal law dictates that a student who is receiving special education services in the public school system must be provided with "transition services" to help facilitate the move between high school and adult life.

It is essential for parents of children with autistic disorders to find out as much as they can concerning the provisions for special educational needs and to consider carefully how to make best use of the services available for their own child. The above information is only a brief outline of some aspects of assessing special educational needs and the legal issues involved. It is always possible that changes will occur, so parents need to make sure they have the latest information. Much more detailed information is available through agencies such as the National Information Center for Children and Youth with Handicaps (NICHCY) and ARC, a national organization providing information and support to individuals with mental retardation and other disabilities. See "The Internet as a Resource" below for website information on these groups.

Occupational Services

Many high-functioning people with autistic disorders can be gainfully employed. A proportion of them settle in jobs that are well below their academic ability and qualifications. This is usually due to their poor social skills and lack of planning ability and flexibility required for higher level occupations. The low level of work may be disappointing to parents, but if it suits the individual concerned, the fact that they are independent should be seen as a success. Disapproval should be avoided so that the self-esteem of the person is not damaged. While employment with non-disabled coworkers is a realistic and appropriate option for some autistic individuals, others may require a job coach to offer needed support. A large proportion of adults with autistic disorders are unable to work in open employment even with support; they need sheltered occupations. Sheltered employment settings are comprised entirely of individuals with disabilities and are supervised by agency personal or special staff. Staff who work in day centers have a variety of past experience and training. Some are specialists in a particular skill or trade such as woodwork or metalwork and offer autistic individuals specific job skill training in their given area of expertise.

An unknown number of adults, after leaving school, have no form of occupation and stay at home all day, perhaps watching the same videos over and over again or engaging in other repetitive activities. It would be most desirable for more opportunities for sheltered work and other activities to be made available. Apart from all the other advantages, this would reduce to some extent the need for residential care.

The Autism Society of America offers more detailed information for adults with autism who are looking for employment, including recommended books and job posting publications.

Respite Care

Respite care is service that offers parents and caregivers a temporary break from caring for their child with autism. Such breaks can help alleviate some of the pressures of living with a child or adult with an autistic disorder. Local agencies or charitable organizations are able to pay for periods of respite care for children and adults with special needs, and parents can themselves pay for some types of placements if they can afford to do so. Places for short-term care are available in some locales by voluntary groups and privately run residential homes. In practice, financial constraints and shortage of suitable placements limit the use that families can make of this service.

A variety of services are worth investigating. State-by-state listings of respite providers are available online through the ARCH National Respite Network and Resource Center (see "The Internet as a Resource," below). The site also offers a link to listings of summer camps for children with autism and other special needs.

In some areas, a system has been set up for linking families who have children with disabilities with other families willing to provide occasional care, perhaps for a half day, overnight, a weekend or even longer. This can work very well but the disturbed behavior and unusual needs of children with autistic disorders make for problems in finding link families who are able to offer suitable care.

Residential Care for Adults

The most able autistic adults organize their own lives. Others in the more able group can live on their own but need some regular support to make sure that their daily needs are being met and to help solve any problems that may arise. Family members or social workers from local, state or federal government agencies or from voluntary organizations may provide this form of assistance.

Adults with autistic disorders who cannot live independently, many of them never diagnosed, can be found in every type of sheltered accommodation. These include group homes, supervised apartments and institutions. Such housing options may be run by local, state or federal government programs or by voluntary or private organizations. Group homes or institutions sometimes work well if the staff understands autistic impairments and the environment is organized enough to suit the individuals with autistic disorders. Problems arise if there is too little structure and the residents have to do much planning for themselves. Decisions regarding housing arrangements should always reflect the needs of the specific individual.

How to Find and Evaluate Services

Most of the effort involved in finding the right services for children and adults with autistic disorders has to come from the parents. Information and advice is available from the Autism Society of America, which has resources on various residential options as well as a bibliography of relevant books and publications. Many local autism societies and parent support groups can also provide information about what is available regionally. Parents should find out as much as they can from other parents who have experience with different services. They should also obtain information from professionals in the field. For special therapies available from those who work privately, the relevant university programs or associations should be able to provide information on how to find qualified local practitioners.

It is essential for parents to visit schools, homes and other services and to be armed with a list of questions. It is necessary to persevere until the queries are answered satisfactorily. The Autism Society of America provides suggestions for essential questions.

Most parents know their own child better than anyone else. It is very useful for parents, teachers and caregivers to exchange information and to learn from each other. Parents naturally want the best for their child and it is right for them to strive to obtain this. However, it helps to retain a sense of proportion and to avoid making demands on the services that are impossible to meet. Knowing when to apply pressure and when to hold back requires cool judgment, which is difficult to have when strong emotions are involved. In such situations it may help to talk about the problems with someone who is sympathetic but who can also be objective. Some compromises are necessary, but this must not mean that the children and adults with autistic disorders are relegated to a poor quality of life.

Practical Advice for Parents

Parents can learn from books and papers some of the general principles of living and working with children who have autistic disorders, but they need specific advice on how to adapt the ideas to their own child. This can be done most effectively if an experienced adviser regularly visits the child's home and bases suggestions on the child's behavior in their everyday environment and on the resources available to the family.

Many social workers in the social services would like to be able to work with individual families, giving emotional support and practical help, but their other commitments make this difficult or impossible. In some areas, psychologists and other professionals working in the social services for people with learning difficulties do home visits and advise parents, but the resources for such intensive work are extremely limited and insufficient time is available for much effective help to be given.

For parents the main source of support, apart from their own family, is often other parents who are in the same situation. Many towns offer organized support groups for parents of autistic individuals. These groups vary widely with regard to composition and approach. Most are chaired by a parent, but a few are run by professionals or school personnel. While some groups meet at a regularly appointed time on a weekly or monthly basis, others are less formally structured. Groups also vary in focus, some being geared toward a specific population, such as parents of adult children with autism or parents of individuals with Asperger syndrome. Local autism societies can also arrange meetings with speakers who are experienced with the practical problems of care. These formal and informal meetings of groups of parents are one of the most valuable sources of support and help.

For families with children attending special schools, the exchange of information and advice between parents and teachers and cooperation with regard to the child's daily program is well worth the effort involved in organizing regular communication.

The Role of Voluntary Organizations

Voluntary organizations play a special role for families with children who have all kinds of disabilities, and help professionals in the field as well. Parents who are members obtain various kinds of help but many also gain from the satisfaction of working with others to initiate and improve services for their children.

The Internet as a Resource

The advent of the internet has marked a major shift in the resources available to parents seeking information on autism and related disorders. The web can be an excellent tool for learning about diagnostic criteria, interventions, resources, evaluations, parent support groups, legal advice, and a host of other issues related to autistic spectrum disorders. Some websites can put parents in touch with experts across the U.S. and around the world. However, it is important to bear in mind that a wide range of information is posted on the internet and it varies in quality. It pays to be judicious in interpreting information found online, critically investigating sources and looking for scientific backing of any claims. If concerns arise as a result of information gleaned from the internet, a professional opinion should be sought.

The following is a list of commonly used websites that provide a range of information on autism and related disorders. These sites also offer links to hundreds of other relevant websites:

ARCH National Respite Network and Resource Center
  www.chtop.com/locator.htm

Asperger Syndrome Coalition of the United States, Inc. (ASC–US)
  www.asperger.org

Autism Resources
  Includes an extensive listing of books relevant to autism
  www.autism-resources.com

Autism Society of America (ASA)
  www.autism-society.org

Birth to Three
  State-by-state contact information for programs for children under age three
  www.birth23.org/Programs/OtherStates.asp

Cure Autism Now (CAN)
  www.canfoundation.org

National Alliance for Autism Research (NAAR)
  www.naar.org

National Information Center for Children and Youth with Handicaps
  Offers legal information
  www.nichcy.org

National Organization of Mental Retardation (ARC)
  www.thearc.org

O.A.S.I.S. (Online Asperger Syndrome Information and Support)
  www.udel.edu/bkirby/asperger

Yale Child Study Center—Developmental Disabilities Clinic and Research Home Page
  www.autism.fm

Postscript

Those of us who live and/or work with children and adults with autistic disorders have to try to enter their world, since they cannot find their way into ours. We need to learn to comprehend and empathize with autistic experiences in order to find ways to help each individual cope with a system of social rules that is alien to them. The reward for the effort involved is a deeper understanding of human social interaction and an appreciation of the wonder of child development. The key to autism is the key to the nature of human life.

Addresses of local autistic societies can be obtained from the Autism Society of America (ASA) headquarters in Maryland or from their website.

Autism Society of America
7910 Woodmont Avenue, Suite 300
Bethesda, MD 20814-3067
Phone: 301-657-0881 or 800-3AUTISM
Fax: 301-657-0869
www.autism-society.org
info@autism-society.org

Reading List

Books

So many interesting and useful books have now been published concerning autistic spectrum disorders and related subjects that it is impossible to give an exhaustive list. The titles mentioned here include all the books referred to in the text together with a few others covering the same topics.

Practical Guidance

Aarons, M. and Gittens, T. *The Handbook of Autism: A Guide for Parents and Professionals*, 2nd ed. London: Routledge, 1999.
> Information on causes, diagnosis, education, development of communication and an objective view of "alternative treatments."

Attwood, T. *Asperger's Syndrome: A Guide for Parents and Professionals*. London: Jessica Kingsley, 1998.
> Helpful discussions of everyday problems and useful, practical suggestions for alleviating them.

Carr, J. *Helping Your Handicapped Child*, 2nd ed. Harmondsworth, Middlesex: Penguin Books, 1995.
> Practical guidance for parents of children with learning difficulties.

Hamilton, L. M. *Facing Autism: Giving Parents Reasons for Hope and Guidance for Help*. Colorado Springs, Colorado: WaterBrook Press, 2000.

Offers advice and guidance for dealing with autism, and provides information on therapies and interventions.

Harris, S. *Siblings of Children with Autism: A Guide for Families.* Bethesda, MD: Woodbine House, 1994.
> Helps parents explain autism to siblings. Gives siblings a chance to share their thoughts and feelings about how their family is different. Practical advice on how children can share time together.

Howlin, P. *Autism in Adolescents and Adults.* London: Routledge, 1996.
> Practical advice, mainly concerned with the more-able adolescents and adults, including those with Asperger's syndrome.

Jordan, R. and Powell, S. *Understanding and Teaching Children with Autism.* Chichester: Wiley, 1995.
> Theory and practice of teaching children with autistic disorders.

McKernan, T. and Mortlock, J. *Autism Focus.* St. Leonards on Sea: Outset Publishing, 1995.
> A training manual for staff working with adults with autistic disorders.

Morgan, H. *Adults with Autism.* Cambridge: Cambridge University Press, 1996.
> Proposals for models of good practice in the services for adults with autistic disorders.

Clinical Descriptions, Research and Theories

Baron-Cohen, S. *Mindblindness: An Essay on Autism and Theory of Mind.* London: MIT, 1995.
> An interesting discussion of the development of "theory of mind" in children and the implications for understanding autism.

Baron-Cohen, S. and Bolton, P. *Autism: The Facts.* London: Oxford University Press, 1994.
> A clear explanation of autism for parents and caregivers.

Frith, U. *Autism: Explaining the Enigma.* Oxford: Blackwell, 1992.
> Ideas on the nature of autism based on results of psychological research.

Frith, U., ed. *Autism and Asperger Syndrome*. Cambridge: Cambridge University Press, 1991.
> Chapters by different authors on the nature of Asperger's syndrome and its relationship to Kanner's autism and other autistic spectrum disorders. A translation into English of Asperger's first paper on his syndrome is included.

Happé, F. *Autism: An Introduction to Psychological Theory*. Cambridge: Harvard University Press, 1998.
> A clear discussion of theories concerning the psychological impairments in autism.

Kanner, L. *Childhood Psychosis: Initial Studies and New Insights*. Washington, DC: Winston, 1973.
> A collection of Kanner's papers on autism, including the original one in which he described 11 children with the typical syndrome. The sequence of papers shows the development of and changes in Kanner's ideas on the subject.

Individual Histories

Grandin, T. and Scariano, M. M. *Emergence: Labeled Autistic*. New York: Warner Books, 1996.
> The life story of a woman with autism who has become independent and runs her own successful business.

Park, C. C. *The Siege*. London: Little, Brown, 1990.
> An account of her daughter's development by the mother of a more-able young woman with autism.

Special Skills in Individuals with Autistic Disorders

Selfe, L. *Nadia: A Case of Extraordinary Drawing Ability in an Autistic Child*. London: Academic Press, 1977.
> The drawings of a young child with autism and a discussion of the nature of her special skill.

Treffert, D. A. *Extraordinary People: Understanding Savant Syndrome*. iUniverse.com, 2000.
> Case histories and discussions of people with remarkable special skills in music, art, calendar calculation, etc.

Wiltshire, S. *Cities*. London: Dent, 1989.
> The detailed architectural drawings of a boy with autism.

The Myths of "Wolf" Children

Clarke, A. M. and Clarke, A. D. B., eds. *Early Experience: Myth and Evidence*. London: Open Books, 1976.
> Case histories and scientific discussions of the effects of early experiences, including isolation from others from an early age.

——*Early Experience and the Life Path*. London: Jessica Kingsley, 2000.

Lane, H. *The Wild Boy of Aveyron*. Cambridge: Harvard University Press, 1979.
> Translations of J. M. G. Itard's reports on Victor, the "wild boy," and an account of the way Itard's methods of teaching Victor have influenced development of education for those with hearing impairments or learning difficulties. Victor's behavior was that of a child with typical autism, although the author of this book did not recognize this!

Causes and Neuropathology

Bauman, M. and Kemper, T., eds. *The Neurobiology of Autism*. Baltimore: Johns Hopkins, 1997.
> Current research in many aspects of the biological basis of autism.

Gillberg, C. and Coleman, M. *The Biology of the Autistic Syndromes*, 3rd ed. London: Mac Keith Press, 2000.
> An overview of the many biological conditions that can be associated with autistic disorders and the medical aspects of investigation and treatment.

Sacks, O. *Awakenings*. New York: Vintage Books, 1999.
> An account of the victims of the epidemic of *encephalitis lethargica* following World War I and their treatment with anti-Parkinson medication. The overlap with the behavior seen in autistic disorders is striking and suggests that the neuropathologies of the two conditions are related.

International Diagnostic Criteria

American Psychiatric Association. *Diagnostic and Statistical Manual*. Washington, DC: APA. DSM III, 1980; DSM III-R, 1987; DSM IV, 1994.

World Health Organization. *International Statistical Classification of Diseases and Related Health Problems*. Geneva: WHO. ICD-8, 1967; ICD-9, 1977; ICD-10, 1992.

World Health Organization. The *ICD-10 Classification of Mental and Behavioral Disorders: Diagnostic Criteria for Research*. Geneva: WHO, 1993.

> These manuals give the diagnostic criteria decided on by committees of professional workers in the field. They are useful for comparative research and statistics but each edition inevitably lags behind the most advanced thinking in the field so should not be used rigidly as a basis for clinical diagnosis and decisions about services needed by individuals.

The "TEACCH" Series

Eric Schopler and Gary Mesibov of the TEACCH Division of the University of North Carolina, Chapel Hill, have edited a series of multi-authored books on many different aspects of autistic spectrum disorders. Further volumes will be published in the future. They are mainly directed at professional workers but are of interest to parents.

The TEACCH division also runs courses on their method of structured and organized education and occupational training. These take place in many different countries.

References to Papers

It is not possible, for reasons of space, to give references to all the papers in the medical, psychological and educational literature relevant to the material in this book. The following list includes only the work of authors specifically mentioned in the text.

Asperger, H. "Die autistischen psychopathen im kindesalter." *Archiv für Psychiatrie und Nervenkrankheiten* 117 (1944): 76–136.

Asperger, H. "Problems of infantile autism." *Communication* 113 (1979): 45–52.

Baron-Cohen, S., Cox, A., Baird, G., Swettenham, J., Nightingale, N., Morgan, K., Drew, A., and Charman, T. "Psychological markers in the detection of autism in infancy in a large population." *British Journal of Psychiatry* (1996).

Bolton, P., MacDonald, H., Pickles, A., Rios, P., Goode, S., Crowson, M., Bailey, A., and Rutter, M. "A case-control family history study of autism." *Journal of Child Psychology and Psychiatry* 35 (1994): 877–900.

Bowler, B. "'Theory of mind' in Asperger's syndrome." *Journal of Child Psychology and Psychiatry* 33 (1994): 877–894.

Ehlers, S. and Gillberg, C. "The epidemiology of Asperger syndrome: A total population study." *Journal of Child Psychology and Psychiatry* 34 (1993): 1327–1350.

Gillberg, C. "Psychotic behavior in children and young adults in a mental handicap hostel." *Acta Psychiatrica Scandinavica* 68 (1983): 351–358.

Gillberg, C. "The Emmanuel Miller Memorial Lecture 1991. Autism and autistic-like conditions: subclasses among disorders of empathy." *Journal of Child Psychology and Psychiatry* 33 (1992): 813–842.

Gillberg, C., Persson, E., Grufman, M. and Themner, U. "Psychiatric disorders in mildly and severely mentally retarded urban children and adolescents: epidemiological aspects." *British Journal of Psychiatry* 149 (1986): 68–74.

Gillberg, C., Rasmussen, P., Carlstrom, G., Svenson, B., and Waldenstrom, E. "Perceptual, motor and attentional deficits in six-year-old children: epidemiological aspects." *Journal of Child Psychology and Psychiatry* 12 (1982): 131–144.

Gillberg, I. C. and Gillberg, C. "Asperger syndrome: some epidemiological considerations." *Journal of Child Psychology and Psychiatry* 30 (1989): 631–638.

Gray, C. "Teaching children with autism to read social situations." In *Teaching Children with Autism Strategies to Enhance Communication and Socialization*, ed. K. A. Quille. London: International Thomson Publications, 1995.

Haslam, J. "Cases of insane children." *Observations on Madness and Melancholy*. London: Haydon (1809): 185–206.

Howlin, P. "The home treatment of autistic children." In *Language and Language Disorders in Children*, eds. L. A. Hersov, M. Berger, and R. Nichol. Oxford: Pergamon Press, 1980.

Kanner, L. "Autistic disturbances of affective contact." *Nervous Child* 2 (1943): 217–250.

Kanner, L. "Irrelevant and metaphorical language in early infantile autism." *American Journal of Psychiatry* 103 (1946): 242–246.

Kolvin, I. "Studies in the childhood psychoses: 1. Diagnostic criteria and classification." *British Journal of Psychiatry* 118 (1971): 381–384.

Lister Brook, S., and Bowler, D. "Autism by another name? Semantic and pragmatic impairments in children." *Journal of Autism and Developmental Disorders* 22 (1992): 61–82.

Maudsley, H. "Insanity of early life." In *The Physiology and Pathology of the Mind*. New York: Appleton (1867): 259–293.

Newson, E. "Pathological demand-avoidance syndrome." *Communication* 17 (1983): 3–8.

Oliver, C. "Self-injurious behavior: from response to strategy." In *Research to Practice? Implications of Research on the Challenging Behavior of People with Learning Disability*, ed. C. Kiernon. Clevedon: BILD, 1993.

Rutter, M. "Concepts of autism: a review of research." *Journal of Child Psychology and Psychiatry* 9 (1968): 1–25.

Tantam, D. "Lifelong eccentricity and social isolation: 1. Psychiatric, social and forensic aspects." *British Journal of Psychiatry* 153 (1988): 777–782.

Wing, L. "The definition and prevalence of autism: a review." *European Child and Adolescent Psychiatry* 2 (1993): 61–74.

Wing, L. and Gould, J. "Severe impairments of social interaction and associated abnormalities in children: epidemiology and classification." *Journal of Autism and Childhood Schizophrenia* 9 (1979): 11–29.

Witmer, L. "Don: A curable case of arrested development due to a fear psychosis in a three-year-old infant." *Psychological Clinics* 13 (1919–22): 97–111.

Index

Other Ulysses Press Mind/Body Titles

HERBS THAT WORK:
THE SCIENTIFIC EVIDENCE OF THEIR HEALING POWERS
David Armstrong, $12.95
Unlike herb books relying on folklore or vague anecdotes, *Herbs that Work* is the first consumer guide to rate herbal remedies based on documented, state-of-the-art scientific research.

HOW MEDITATION HEALS: A SCIENTIFIC EXPLANATION
Eric Harrison, $12.95
In straightforward, practical terms, *How Meditation Heals* reveals how and why meditation improves the natural functioning of the human body.

HOW TO MEDITATE: AN ILLUSTRATED GUIDE
TO CALMING THE MIND AND RELAXING THE BODY
Paul Roland, $16.95
Offers a friendly, illustrated approach to calming the mind and raising consciousness through various techniques, including basic meditation, visualization, body scanning for tension, affirmations and mantras.

THE JOSEPH H. PILATES METHOD AT HOME:
A BALANCE, SHAPE, STRENGTH & FITNESS PROGRAM
Eleanor McKenzie, $16.95
This handbook describes and details Pilates, a mental and physical program that combines elements of yoga and classical dance.

KNOW YOUR BODY: THE ATLAS OF ANATOMY
2nd edition, Introduction by Emmet B. Keeffe, M.D., $14.95
Provides a comprehensive, full-color guide to the human body.

101 SIMPLE WAYS TO MAKE YOUR HOME & FAMILY
SAFE IN A TOXIC WORLD
Beth Ann Petro Roybal, $9.95
Sheds light on common toxins found around the house and offers parents straightforward ways to protect themselves and their children.

PILATES WORKBOOK: ILLUSTRATED STEP-BY-STEP GUIDE
TO MATWORK TECHNIQUES
Michael King, $12.95
Illustrates the core matwork movements exactly as Joseph Pilates intended them to be performed; readers learn each movement by simply following the photographic sequences and explanatory captions.

SENSES WIDE OPEN:
THE ART AND PRACTICE OF LIVING IN YOUR BODY
Johanna Putnoi, $14.95
Through simple, accessible exercises, this book shows how to be at ease with yourself and experience genuine pleasure in your physical connection to others and the world.

THE 7 HEALING CHAKRAS:
UNLOCKING YOUR BODY'S ENERGY CENTERS
Brenda Davies, $14.95
Explores the essence of chakras, vortices of energy that connect the physical body with the spiritual.

SIMPLY RELAX: AN ILLUSTRATED GUIDE
TO SLOWING DOWN AND ENJOYING LIFE
Dr. Sarah Brewer, $15.95
In a beautifully illustrated format, this book clearly presents physical and mental disciplines that show readers how to relax.

TEACH YOURSELF TO MEDITATE IN 10 SIMPLE LESSONS: DISCOVER RELAXATION AND CLARITY OF MIND IN JUST MINUTES A DAY
Eric Harrison, $12.95
Guides the reader through ten easy-to-follow core meditations. Also included are practical and enjoyable "spot meditations" that require only a few minutes a day and can be incorporated into the busiest of schedules.

WEEKEND HOME SPA: FOUR CREATIVE ESCAPES—
CLEANSING, ENERGIZING, RELAXING AND PAMPERING
Linda Bird, $16.95
Shows how to create that spa experience in your own home with step-by-step mini workouts, stretching routines, meditations and visualizations, as well as more challenging exercises to boost mental potential.

To order these books call 800-377-2542 or 510-601-8301, fax 510-601-8307, e-mail ulysses@ulyssespress.com, or write to Ulysses Press, P.O. Box 3440, Berkeley, CA 94703. All retail orders are shipped free of charge. California residents must include sales tax. Allow two to three weeks for delivery.

About the Author

An internationally recognized medical authority, Dr. Lorna Wing has been studying autism for 30 years. She is also the mother of an autistic daughter. Her work with autistic children in the 1970s redefined the classic profile of autism and helped create the concept of autistic spectrum disorders. Throughout her career, Dr. Wing has developed practical and constructive ways for parents to cope with the wide range of difficulties experienced by families caring for autistic children. She is the psychiatric consultant for the National Autistic Society in the United Kingdom and her numerous books and papers have been translated into several languages. She lives in East Sussex, England.